Math for Nurses

A Pocket Guide to Dosage Calculation and Drug Preparation

Second Edition

Math for Nurses

A Pocket Guide to Dosage Calculation and Drug Preparation
Second Edition

Mary Jo Boyer, M.S.N.

Assistant Dean of Allied Health &
Director of Nursing
Delaware County Community College
Media, Pennsylvania

Marie Clark, M.S.N.
Consultant

J. B. Lippincott Company

Philadelphia
New York ■ St. Louis
London ■ Sydney ■ Tokyo

Sponsoring Editor: Ellen M. Campbell
Project Coordinator: Lori J. Bainbridge
Production: Editorial Services of New England, Inc.
Compositor: Publication Services, Inc.
Printer/Binder: R. R. Donnelly & Sons Company

Second Edition

6 5 4 3

Library of Congress Cataloging-in-Publication Data

Boyer, Mary Jo.
  Math for nurses: a pocket guide to dosage calculation and drug
preparation/Mary Jo Boyer : Marie Clark, consultant.
    p. cm.
  Includes index.
  ISBN 0-397-54828-1
  1. Nursing—Mathematics—Handbooks, manuals, etc.
2. Pharmaceutical arithmetic—Handbooks, manuals, etc. I. Clark,
Marie, 1943-. II. Title.
  [DNLM 1. Dosage Forms—handbooks.   2. Dosage Forms—nurse's
instruction.   3. Mathematics—handbooks.   4. Mathematics—nurse's
instruction.   5. Pharmacology—handbooks.   6. Pharmacology—nurse's
instruction.   QV 735 B791m]
RT88.B68   1990
615'. 14—dc20
DNLM/DLC
for Library of Congress   90-6489
                                                              CIP

Any procedure or practice described in this book should be applied by the health-care practitioner under appropriate supervision in accordance with professional standards of care used with regard to the unique circumstances that apply in each practice situation. Care has been taken to confirm the accuracy of information presented and to describe generally accepted practices. However, the authors, editors, and publisher cannot accept any responsibility for errors or omissions or for any consequences from application of the information in this book and make no warranty, express or implied, with respect to the contents of the book.

Every effort has been made to ensure drug selections and dosages are in accordance with current recommendations and practice. Because of ongoing research, changes in government regulations and the constant flow of information on drug therapy, reactions and interactions, the reader is cautioned to check the package insert for each drug for indications, dosages, warnings and precautions, particularly if the drug is new or infrequently used.

To my parents, Ermelina and John Flynn,
who never stop nurturing.

Preface

The idea for this compact, pocket-sized book about dosage calculation was generated by my students. For several years I watched as they took their math-related handouts and photocopied them, reducing them to a size that would fit into the pockets of their uniform or laboratory coats. This "pocket" reference material was readily accessible when a math calculation was needed to administer a drug. Each year the number of papers that were copied increased as each group of students passed on their ideas to the next group. I also noted that staff nurses were using this readily available and compact information as a reference for math problems.

When a student then asked: "Why not put together for us all the information that we need?" I thought, "Why not?" The idea was born, the commitment made, and 12 months later the first edition of MATH FOR NURSES was finished. It is my hope that it will continue, in this new edition, to be helpful to all who need a quick reference source when struggling with dosage calculation and drug preparation.

This pocket guide is divided into three units to facilitate quick access to specific information needed to administer drugs. Unit I presents a review of basic math, starting with the fundamentals of Roman and arabic numerals. Chapters 2 and 3 cover fractions and decimals. Chapter 4 shows you how to set up a ratio and proportion and solve for *x*, using a colon or fraction format. It also uses drug-related word problems as examples to help you solve for *x*. This information is essential—a foundation for understanding the dosage calculations presented in Unit III.

Unit II focuses on the metric system, the apothecaries' system, and household units of measurement. Chapter 8 lists system equivalents and shows you how to convert from one unit of measurement to another. The system equivalents on page 111 are duplicated on the inside front cover to provide easy and quick access when calculating drug problems.

Unit III is the most comprehensive and detailed section of this pocket guide. The chapters cover oral and parenteral dosage problems. There is a separate section on vaccines, toxoids, and immune serum globulins, as well as a section addressing pediatric and geriatric considerations. Intravenous fluid therapy is discussed, along with the preparation and administration of solutions. Throughout this unit, problem-solving methodology is presented in a simple, easy-to-follow manner. A step-by-step approach is used, which will guide the reader through each set of examples.

Every chapter ends with a series of practice problems, and a full set of appendices (eight) provide the necessary supplemental information needed to understand and master preparation of medications.

MATH FOR NURSES was written for all nurses who administer drugs. It is intended as a quick, easy, and readily accessible guide when dosage calculations are required. It is my hope that its use will help nurses to calculate dosages accurately and, as a result, to improve the accuracy of drug delivery.

It is our inherent responsibility as nurses to ensure that every patient entrusted to our care receives the correct dosage of medication delivered in the most appropriate way.

Mary Jo Boyer, R.N., M.S.N.

How to Use This Book

This book is designed for two purposes:

- To help you learn how to calculate drug dosages and administer medications.
- To serve as a quick reference when reinforcement of learning is required.

The best way to use this pocket guide is to:

- Read the rules and examples.
- Follow the steps for solving the problems.
- Work the practice problems.
- Write down your answers and notes in the margin so you have a quick reference when you need to review.

Contents

Math for Nurses

A Pocket Guide to Dosage Calculation and Drug Preparation

Second Edition

Unit 1

Basic Mathematics Review

This unit presents a basic review of Roman numerals, fractions, decimals, and ratio-proportion. Chapter 1 gives an overview of Roman numerals and their Arabic equivalents. The ability to solve for x assumes a basic mastery of fractions and decimals. Therefore a brief review of addition, subtraction, multiplication, and division for fractions and decimals has been provided in Chapters 2 and 3 so that you can review this material. In order to calculate accurately dosage problems, you need to be able to transcribe a word problem into a mathematical equation. This process is presented in a "step-by-step" format in Chapter 4.

Chapter 1

Roman Numerals with Arabic Equivalents

In the Arabic system numerals (1 to 10) are used to express quantity or measure. The Arabic system lends itself nicely to the use of fractions and decimals, as well as to the basic mathematical exercises of addition, subtraction, multiplication, and division.

The use of Roman numerals dates back to ancient times, when those in the medical profession used its symbols for pharmaceutical computations and record keeping. Modern medicine has retained some of that tradition by using Roman numerals in prescribing medications. This tradition is also evident in the apothecaries' system of weights and measurement, which consistently uses Roman numerals.

The Roman system uses letters to designate numbers; the most commonly used letters can be found in Table 1–1. Four numerals are rarely used in practice (50, 100, 500, 1000) but are included in the table for your review.

The Roman numeral system follows certain rules for arrangement of its numerals.

■ RULE: **To Write Roman Numerals, Follow These Steps:**

- Place the *largest*-valued numerals on the *left*.

Table 1–1. Roman Numeral Equivalents for Arabic Numerals

ARABIC NUMERAL	ROMAN NUMERAL
1/2	ss
1	i
2	ii
3	iii
4	iv
5	v
6	vi
7	vii
8	viii
9	ix
10	x
15	xv
20	xx
30	xxx
50	L
100	C
500	D
1000	M

■ Place the *smallest*-valued numerals on the *right*.

EXAMPLES: 15   xv
25   xxv

■ **RULE: To Read Roman Numerals, Follow This Step:**

■ The smallest-valued numerals on the right are *added to* the largest-valued numerals on the left.

EXAMPLES: xv $10 + 5 = 15$
             xxiii $20 + 3 = 23$

■ **RULE: To Repeat Roman Numerals, Follow This Step:**

- Roman numerals of the same value can be repeated in sequence, *only up to three times*. Once you can no longer repeat, you need to subtract.

EXAMPLES: $4 = 5 \text{ (v)} - 1 \text{ (i)} = \text{iv}$
             $9 = 10 \text{ (x)} - 1 \text{ (i)} = \text{ix}$
             $40 = 50 \text{ (L)} - 10 \text{ (x)} = \text{XL}$

NOTE: Three numerals *may never be repeated* in sequence because their value, when doubled, becomes a separate Roman numeral. These are L, v, and D.

EXAMPLES: C   100   *not* LL
             x   10   *not* vv
             M   1000   *not* DD

Practice Problems

Change the following Arabic numerals to Roman numerals:

1. 1/2 _____   4. 10 _____

2. 3 _____   5. 15 _____

3. 7 _____   6. 30 _____

Change the following Roman numerals to Arabic numerals:

7. vi _____   10. ix _____

8. ii _____   11. xx _____

9. v _____   12. xxv _____

End of Chapter Review

Write the following Arabic numerals as Roman numerals:

1. 27   *Answer =*

2. 32   *Answer =*

3. 16   *Answer =*

4. 4   *Answer =*

5. 8   *Answer =*

6. 10   *Answer =*

7. 12   *Answer =*

8. 21   *Answer =*

9. 18   *Answer =*

10. 24   *Answer =*

Write the following numerals as Arabic numerals:

11. xviii   *Answer* =

12. xvi   *Answer* =

13. ss   *Answer* =

14. ix   *Answer* =

15. viiss   *Answer* =

16. xix   *Answer* =

17. xxiv   *Answer* =

18. xiv   *Answer* =

19. xxvi   *Answer* =

20. vi   *Answer* =

Chapter 2

Fractions

Many drug preparations are prescribed and prepared in fractions. You will need to know how to calculate drug dosages when fractions are used.

A *fraction* is a portion or piece of a whole that indicates division of that whole into equal units or parts. For example, if you divide an apple into four equal parts, each part is considered to be 1/4 of the apple. Each section is a fraction of the apple.

Fractions are made up of a numerator and a denominator. The top number of the fraction is the numerator and the bottom number is the denominator. Look at the example below:

$$\text{Fraction} = \frac{3}{4} = \frac{\text{numerator}}{\text{denominator}}$$

For the fraction $\frac{3}{4}$, 3 is the numerator and 4 is the denominator.

Remember the following rule:

■ RULE: **The Numerator is the Number on the *Top* of the Fraction and the Denominator is the Number on the *Bottom* of the Fraction.**

Practice Problems

For the fractions below, place an "N" next to the numerator and a "D" next to the denominator.

1. $\frac{4}{5}$ 4. $\frac{4}{9}$

2. $\frac{1}{2}$ 5. $\frac{7}{8}$

3. $\frac{3}{8}$ 6. $\frac{1}{6}$

The Denominator of a Fraction

The denominator of a fraction tells you the number of equal parts into which the whole has been divided. For example, if you divide something into 4 equal parts, each part would be expressed as a fraction that has the denominator of 4. That is, each part would be equal to 1/4. If you divide something into eight equal parts, the denominator would be 8, and each part would be equal to 1/8. Look at Figure 2–1, which illustrates two circles: one is divided into fourths and one is divided into eighths.

If you look at the circles, you will notice that the circle that is divided into 1/8's has smaller portions than the circle that is divided into 1/4's. The reason is that the *fraction 1/8 is less than 1/4.* Even though 1/8 has a larger denominator (8) than 1/4 (4), it is a smaller fraction. This is an important concept to understand: that is, the bigger the

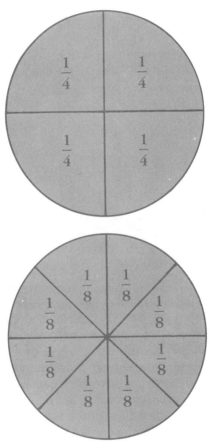

Figure 2-1. Two circles: the whole divided into equal parts.

number in the denominator, the smaller the fraction or pieces of the whole. To clarify, consider these examples:

$$\frac{1}{2} \text{ is greater than } \frac{1}{4}$$

$$\frac{1}{8} \text{ is greater than } \frac{1}{16}$$

$$\frac{1}{9} \text{ is greater than } \frac{1}{10}$$

Remember the following rule:

■ **RULE: The Bigger the Number in the Denominator, the Smaller the Pieces (or Fractions) of the Whole.**

Practice Problems

Arrange the fractions below in order of size. That is, list the *smallest fraction first*, then the next smallest fraction, and so on until you finish by listing the *largest fraction last*.

$$\frac{1}{9} \quad \frac{1}{12} \quad \frac{1}{3} \quad \frac{1}{7} \quad \frac{1}{150} \quad \frac{1}{25} \quad \frac{1}{100} \quad \frac{1}{300} \quad \frac{1}{75}$$

The Numerator of a Fraction

The numerator tells you how many of the equal parts you have. For example, the numerator 2 in the fraction 2/3 tells you that you have *two* equal parts that are each worth 1/3. The numerator 3 in the fraction 3/5 tells you that you have *three* equal parts that are each worth 1/5.

Practice Problems

Look at the first example problem below. Then fill in the blanks in the rest.

1. 7/8 means that you have __7__ equal parts worth __1/8__ each.

2. 9/10 means that you have _____ equal parts worth _____ each.

3. 4/5 means that you have _____ equal parts worth _____ each.

4. 23/25 means that you have _____ equal parts worth _____ each.

5. 4/150 means that you have _____ equal parts worth _____ each.

Fractions That Are Equal to One, More Than One, or Less Than One

The rules below tell you how to decide if a fraction is equal to one, more than one, or less than one.

■ RULE: **If the Numerator and Denominator Are Equal to Each Other, the Fraction Is Equal to One.**

EXAMPLES: $\frac{1}{1} = 1$, $\frac{3}{3} = 1$, $\frac{25}{25} = 1$

$$\frac{125}{125} = 1, \quad \frac{325}{325} = 1$$

■ RULE: If the Numerator is *Greater Than* the Denominator, the Fraction Is Equal to More Than One.

EXAMPLES: $\frac{2}{1} = 2, \quad \frac{5}{4} = 1\frac{1}{4}, \quad \frac{3}{2} = 1\frac{1}{2}$

■ RULE: If the Numerator is *Less Than* the Denominator, the Fraction Is Equal to Less Than One. (The Symbol < Means Less Than One.)

EXAMPLES: $\frac{3}{4} < 1, \quad \frac{7}{8} < 1, \quad \frac{9}{10} < 1$

Mixed Numbers and Improper Fractions

Fractions that are equal to more than one may be written in two ways: as mixed numbers or as improper fractions.

Mixed Numbers consist of a whole number *and* a fraction written together.

EXAMPLES: $1\frac{1}{2}, \quad 3\frac{3}{4}, \quad 5\frac{4}{5}$

Improper Fractions are fractions that have a numerator greater than the denominator.

EXAMPLES: $\frac{3}{2},\quad \frac{15}{4},\quad \frac{29}{5}$

Mixed numbers can be changed to improper fractions. For example, 1 1/2 can be changed to 3/2. The following rule tells you how to change a mixed number to an improper fraction.

Changing a Mixed Number to an Improper Franction

■ **RULE: To Change a Mixed Number to an Improper Fraction Follow These Steps:**

- Multiply the denominator of the fraction by the whole number. That is, if you have the fraction of 2 3/4, you would multiply 2 × 4, which equals 8.
- Add the numerator of the fraction (3) to the answer you got when you multiplied the denominator by the whole number in the above step (8). Using the example above, this means that you would add 3 to 8, and get the answer of 11.
- The answer that you got in the above step (11) becomes the new numerator of the new single fraction. The denominator in the original mixed fraction (which is 4 in this example) stays the same.

The *mixed number* 2 3/4 becomes the *improper fraction* 11/4.

Practice Problems

Change the following mixed numbers to improper fractions:

1. $5\frac{9}{12}$

Answer =

2. $6\frac{7}{8}$

Answer =

3. $8\frac{3}{5}$

Answer =

4. $15\frac{1}{9}$

Answer =

5. $32\frac{2}{3}$

Answer =

6. $21\frac{3}{4}$

Answer =

7. $18\frac{1}{2}$

Answer =

8. $6\frac{3}{9}$

Answer =

9. $5\frac{2}{5}$

Answer =

10. $11\frac{1}{6}$

Answer =

Improper fractions can also be changed to mixed numbers. For example, the fraction 5/4 can be changed to 1 1/4. Often, when you are working the mathematics for a given problem, you will need to work with improper fractions. However, if you get a final answer that is an improper fraction, convert it to a mixed number. For example, it is better to say "I have 1 1/4 apples" than to say "I have 5/4 apples." Look at the rule below which tells you how to change an improper fraction to a mixed number.

Changing an Improper Fraction to a Mixed Number

■ **Rule: To Change an Improper Fraction to a Mixed Number, Follow these Steps:**

- Divide the top number (numerator) by the bottom number (denominator). If you use the example of 13/7, this means you would divide 13 by 7:

$$7)\overline{13} \begin{array}{r} 1 \\ \underline{7} \\ 6 \end{array} \text{ leftover}$$

- The number that you get when you divide the numerator by the denominator becomes the whole number of the mixed number. In the above example, (1) becomes the whole number.

- The number that you have left over (6 in the example above) becomes the numerator of the fraction that goes with the whole number to make it a mixed number. Using the above example, your answer would look like this so far: 1 6/?

- The *original* denominator of the fraction of the mixed number (which is 7 in this case) becomes the denominator of the fraction of

the mixed number. In this example, the improper fraction, 13/7, becomes the mixed
number, 1 6/7.

Practice Problems

Change the following improper fractions to mixed
numbers:

1. $\dfrac{30}{4}$

Answer =

2. $\dfrac{41}{6}$

Answer =

3. $\dfrac{68}{9}$

Answer =

4. $\dfrac{72}{11}$

Answer =

5. $\dfrac{90}{12}$

Answer =

6. $\dfrac{40}{15}$

Answer =

7. $\dfrac{86}{20}$

Answer =

8. $\dfrac{62}{8}$

Answer =

9. $\dfrac{86}{9}$

Answer =

10. $\dfrac{112}{5}$

Answer =

Equivalent or Equal Fractions

Changing Fractions with Different Denominators to Equivalent or Equal Fractions

When you are working problems with fractions, it is sometimes necessary to change a fraction to a different but equivalent fraction. For example, it may be necessary to change 2/4 to 1/2 or 2/3 to 4/6. You can make a new fraction that has the same value by either multiplying or dividing *both* the numerator and the denominator by the *same* number. Look at the examples below.

EXAMPLES: $\frac{2}{3}$ can be changed to $\frac{4}{6}$ by multiplying both the numerator and the denominator by 2.

$$\left(\frac{2 \times 2 = 4}{3 \times 2 = 6}\right)$$

$\frac{2}{4}$ can be changed to $\frac{1}{2}$ by dividing both the numerator and the denominator by 2.

$$\left(\frac{2 \div 2 = 1}{4 \div 2 = 2}\right)$$

It is important to remember that you can change the numerator and the denominator of a fraction and still keep the same value *so long as you follow the following rule*:

■ RULE: **When Changing a Fraction, You Must Do the Same Thing (Multiply or Divide by the Same Number) to the Numerator and to the Denominator in Order to Keep the Same Value.**

EXAMPLES: To change the fraction $\frac{4}{5}$ to $\frac{8}{10}$

multiply 4×2 and 5×2.

$$\left(\frac{4 \times 2 = 8}{5 \times 2 = 10}\right)$$

$\frac{4}{5}$ has the same value as $\frac{8}{10}$

To change the fraction $\frac{4}{16}$ to $\frac{1}{4}$

divide 4 by 4 and 16 by 4.

$$\left(\frac{4 \div 4 = 1}{16 \div 4 = 4}\right)$$

$\frac{4}{16}$ has the same value as $\frac{1}{4}$

To determine that both fractions have equal value, multiply the opposite numerators and denominators. For example, if $4/5 = 8/10$, then the product of 4×10 will equal the product of 5×8.

$$4 \times 10 = 40 \quad \text{and} \quad 5 \times 8 = 40$$

Practice Problems

1. 3/5 is equivalent to: 6/15 or 9/10 or 12/20.

   Answer =

2. 4/8 is equivalent to: 8/24 or 12/16 or 20/40.

   Answer =

3. 6/12 is equivalent to: 2/4 or 3/5 or 12/36.

   Answer =

4. 10/16 is equivalent to: 20/48 or 5/8 or 30/32.

   Answer =

5. 12/20 is equivalent to: 3/5 or 6/5 or 4/10.

   Answer =

6. 18/30 is equivalent to: 3/15 or 9/10 or 6/10.

   Answer =

7. 9/54 is equivalent to: 3/16 or 1/6 or 1/8.

Answer =

8. 15/90 is equivalent to: 1/6 or 3/8 or 5/14.

Answer =

9. 14/56 is equivalent to: 2/6 or 1/4 or 7/8.

Answer =

10. 8/144 is equivalent to: 2/36 or 4/23 or 1/18.

Answer =

Simplifying, or Reducing, Fractions

It is often easier to work with fractions that have been simplified, or reduced to the lowest terms. This means that the numerator and the denominator are the smallest numbers that can still represent the fraction or piece of the whole. For example, 4/10 can be reduced to 2/5; 4/8 can be reduced to 1/2. It is important to know how to reduce (or simplify) a fraction. The following rule outlines the steps for reducing a fraction to the lowest terms:

■ RULE: **To Reduce a Fraction to its Lowest Terms, Follow These Steps:**

- Study both the numerator and denominator and determine the largest number that can go evenly into *both* the numerator *and* the denominator. For example, suppose you were trying to reduce the fraction 9/18. The largest number that will go into *both* the numerator (9) and the denominator (18) is 9.

- Divide *both* the numerator and the denominator by the number that you determined will go evenly into both of them. Using the example above, this means you would do the following:

$$\frac{9 \div 9}{18 \div 9} = \frac{1}{2}$$

Consider these examples:

$\frac{6}{10}$ can be reduced to $\frac{3}{5}$ by dividing both the numerator and the denominator by 2.

$\frac{5}{15}$ can be reduced to $\frac{1}{3}$ by dividing both the numerator and the denominator by 5.

Practice Problems

Reduce the following fractions to their lowest terms:

1. $\dfrac{8}{48}$

Answer =

2. $\dfrac{6}{36}$

Answer =

3. $\dfrac{4}{36}$

Answer =

Addition of Fractions

Fractions can be added whether the denominators are like (same) or unlike.

Addition of Fractions with Like Denominators

■ **RULE: To Add Fractions with Like Denominators, Follow These Steps:**
   ▪ Add the numerators. For example, to add $1/5 + 3/5$, add the numerators $1 + 3 = 4$.

- Place the new numerator over the like denominator that remains the same. Place 4 over 5 or 4/5.
- Reduce to lowest terms, if necessary.
- Change any improper fraction to a mixed number.

EXAMPLE: $\frac{1}{7} + \frac{4}{7}$

Change: $\frac{1}{7} + \frac{4}{7} = \frac{1}{7} \, \frac{+ \, 4}{7} = \frac{5}{7}$

5 = numerator

7 = like denominator

Answer $= \frac{5}{7}$

EXAMPLE: $\frac{1}{6} + \frac{9}{6}$

Change: $\frac{1}{6} + \frac{9}{6} = \frac{1}{6} \, \frac{+ \, 9}{6} = \frac{10}{6}$

10 = new numerator

6 = like denominator

$\frac{10}{6}$ — needs to be reduced

Reduce: $\frac{10}{6} = \frac{10 \div 2}{6 \div 2} = \frac{5}{3} = \begin{array}{l} \text{improper} \\ \text{fraction} \end{array}$

Change: $\frac{5}{3} = 5 \div 3 = 1\frac{2}{3}$

Answer $= 1\frac{2}{3}$

Addition of Fractions
with Unlike Denominators

■ RULE: **To Add Fractions with Unlike Denominators, Follow These Steps:**

- Find a common denominator. The *easiest way* to find a common denominator is to multiply all the denominators. For example, to add 1/4 + 3/5 find a common denominator by multiplying the denominators 4 × 5 = 20.
- Change the unlike fractions to like fractions.

1. Divide the common denominator of 20 by the denominator of each fraction.

   For the fraction $\frac{1}{4}$,

   $$\text{divide } 4\overline{)20}\ \underline{}\!\!^{5}\text{ (quotient)}$$

   For the fraction $\frac{3}{5}$,

   $$\text{divide } 5\overline{)20}\ \underline{}\!\!^{4}\text{ (quotient)}$$

2. Take each new quotient and multiply it by the numerator of each fraction.

   For the fraction 1/4, multiply the numerator 1 by the quotient 5 for the new numerator of 5.

For the fraction 3/5, multiply the numerator 3 by the quotient 4 for a new numerator of 12.

$$\frac{1}{4} \text{ becomes } \frac{5}{20}$$

$$\frac{3}{5} \text{ becomes } \frac{12}{20}$$

▪ Add the new numerators and place your answer over the common denominator. Reduce to lowest terms if necessary.

$$5 + 12 = 17$$

$$Answer = \frac{17}{20}$$

EXAMPLE: Add $\frac{1}{3} + \frac{5}{6}$.

A common denominator would be 18 (6×3).

$$\text{Change } \frac{1}{3} \text{ to } \frac{6}{18}$$

$$\text{Change } \frac{5}{6} \text{ to } \frac{15}{18}$$

Add the new numerators.

$6 + 15 = 21$ $\frac{21}{18}$ needs to be reduced to $\frac{7}{6}$

$$\frac{7}{6} \text{ should be changed to } 1\frac{1}{6}$$

$$Answer = 1\frac{1}{6}$$

Addition of Mixed Numbers

■ **RULE: To Add Fractions with a Mixed Number, Follow These Steps:**

- Change the mixed number to an improper fraction.
  To add 1/6 + 2 3/8 + 5/6, change 2 3/8 to 19/8.
- Find a common denominator. For the denominators of 6 and 8 the common denominator is 48 (6 × 8).
- Change the unlike fractions to like fractions.

$$\frac{1}{6} \text{ becomes } \frac{8}{48}$$

$$\frac{19}{8} \text{ becomes } \frac{114}{48}$$

$$\frac{5}{6} \text{ becomes } \frac{40}{48}$$

- Add the new numerators and place your answer over the common denominator.

$$8 + 114 + 40 = \frac{162}{48}$$

■ Reduce if necessary.

$$\frac{162}{48} = \frac{27}{8} = 3\frac{3}{8}$$

Answer $= 3\frac{3}{8}$

Subtraction of Fractions

Fractions can be subtracted whose denominators are like (same) or unlike.

Subtraction of Fractions with Like Denominators

■ **RULE: To Subtract Fractions with Like Denominators Subtract the Numerators.**

To subtract fractions with like denominators simply subtract the numerators. If you need to subtract 3/8 from 7/8, simply subract 3 from 7, which equals 4. Place the new numerator 4 over 8 and reduce 4/8 to 1/2.

EXAMPLES: $\frac{5}{6} - \frac{3}{6} = 5 - 3 = 2$

$\frac{2}{6} = \frac{1}{3}$, new fraction

$\frac{7}{8} - \frac{4}{8} = 7 - 4 = 3$

$\frac{3}{8}$, a new fraction

Subtraction of Fractions
with Unlike Denominators

You will probably never need to subtract unlike
fractions or fractions with a mixed number to calculate dosage problems. However, both will be
presented here briefly in case you want to review
the steps.

■ RULE: **To Subtract Fractions
with Unlike Denominators,
Follow These Steps:**

- Find a common denominator. To subtract
  3/5 from 5/6, find the common denominator
  of 30 (6 × 5).
- Change the unlike fractions to like fractions
  (Refer to page 27 to review changing unlike
  fractions to like fractions if you need help.)

$$\frac{5}{6} \text{ becomes } \frac{25}{30}$$

$$\frac{3}{5} \text{ becomes } \frac{18}{30}$$

- Subtract the new numerators and place your
  answer over the common denominator. 25
  − 18 = 7, the numerator. Place 7 over 30,
  7/30.

Answer $= \dfrac{7}{30}$

Subtraction of Mixed Numbers

There are two methods of subtracting mixed numbers:

1. Subtract the fractions by changing the mixed number to an improper fraction. For example, to subtract 3/6 from 2 1/8 you want to change the mixed number (2 1/8) to an improper fraction.

▪ RULE: **To Subtract Fractions with a Mixed Number, Follow These Steps:**

  ▪ Change the mixed number to an improper fraction.
    To subtract 3/6 from 2 1/8 change 2 1/8 to 17/8.
  ▪ Find a common denominator.
    For the denominators 8 and 6 the common denominator is 48 (6 × 8).
  ▪ Change the unlike fractions to like fractions.

$$\frac{17}{8} \text{ becomes } \frac{102}{48}$$

$$\frac{3}{6} \text{ becomes } \frac{24}{48}$$

  ▪ Subtract the new numerators and place your answer over the common denominator. 102 − 24 = 78, the new numerator.

$$\text{Place } \frac{78}{48} = \frac{13}{8} = 1\frac{5}{8}$$

$$Answer = 1\frac{5}{8}$$

2. Subtract the fractions by leaving the mixed number as is. For example, to subtract 3/6 from 2 1/8 you can leave 2 1/8 as is and set up your subtraction like this:

$$2\frac{1}{8}$$
$$-\frac{3}{6}$$

■ **RULE: To Subtract Fractions with a Mixed Number Follow These Steps:**

- Find a common denominator. For the denominators of 6 and 8, the common denominator is 48.
- Change the unlike denominators.

$$2\frac{1}{8} \text{ becomes } 2\ \frac{6}{48}$$

$$\frac{3}{6} \text{ becomes } \frac{24}{48}$$

- Subtract the numerators; subtract the whole numbers.
  Note: To subtract 24/48 from 2 26/48 you need to borrow 1 or 48/48 from the whole number 2. Add 48 to 6 = 54, a new numerator.

EXAMPLE:

$$2\frac{6}{48} = \quad 1\frac{54}{48}$$

$$-\ \frac{24}{48} = -\ \frac{24}{48}$$

$$1\frac{30}{48} = 1\frac{5}{8}$$

Answer $= 1\frac{5}{8}$

Practice Problems

Addition of Fractions

1. $\frac{5}{11} + \frac{9}{11} + \frac{13}{11}$

Answer =

2. $\frac{7}{16} + \frac{3}{8}$

Answer =

3. $\frac{4}{6} + 3\frac{1}{8}$

Answer =

4. $\frac{11}{15} + \frac{14}{45}$

Answer =

5. $\frac{5}{20} + \frac{8}{20} + \frac{13}{20}$

Answer =

Subtraction of Fractions

6. $\frac{6}{7} - \frac{3}{7}$

Answer =

7. $\frac{8}{9} - \frac{4}{9}$

Answer =

8. $\frac{3}{5} - \frac{1}{6}$

Answer =

9. $\frac{3}{4} - \frac{2}{9}$

Answer =

10. $6\frac{3}{7} - \frac{2}{3}$

Answer =

Multiplication of Fractions

Multiplying a Fraction by Another Fraction

Multiplying fractions is easy. All that you have to do is multiply the numerators times each other, and the denominators times each other. For example, if you want to multiply 3/4 × 2/3, you would multiply 3 × 2, to get the new numerator, and 4 × 3, to get the new denominator.

EXAMPLES: $\frac{3}{4} \times \frac{2}{3} = \frac{6}{12}$ or $\frac{1}{2}$ $\frac{1}{2} \times \frac{2}{3} = \frac{2}{6}$ or $\frac{1}{3}$

Remember the following rule for multiplying fractions:

■ **RULE: To Multiply Fractions, Multiply the Numerators to Get the New Numerator, and Multiply the Denominators to Get the New Denominator.**

EXAMPLE: $\frac{1}{5} \times \frac{1}{2} = \frac{1}{10}$

This method of multiplying fractions is sometimes considered to be the "long form" or long method. There is also a "short cut" method for multiplying fractions, called "cancellation." With cancellation, you actually simplify the numbers *before* you multiply. Look at the example below:

EXAMPLE: $\frac{1}{4} \times \frac{8}{15}$

Cancellation can be used because the denominator of the first fraction (4) and the numerator of the second fraction (8) can both be divided by 4. So, if you work the problem, it looks like this:

$$\frac{1}{4} \times \frac{8}{15} = \frac{1}{\cancel{4}_{1}} \times \frac{\cancel{8}^{2}}{15}$$

Once you have cancelled all the numbers that you can, you then multiply the new numerators and the new denominators to get your answer.

$$\frac{1}{1} \times \frac{2}{15} = \frac{2}{15}$$

$$Answer = \frac{2}{15}$$

Multiplying a Fraction by a Mixed Number

Whenever you have to multiply a mixed number, you should always convert it to an improper fraction before you work the problem. Remember the rule:

■ **RULE: To Multiply a Fraction That Involves a Mixed Number, Change the Mixed Number to an Improper Fraction *Before You Work the Problem.***

EXAMPLES:

$$1\frac{1}{2} \times \frac{1}{2}$$

Change $1\frac{1}{2}$ to $\frac{3}{2}$

Multiply $\frac{3}{2} \times \frac{1}{2}$

$$Answer = \frac{3}{4}$$

$$1\frac{1}{2} \times 4\frac{1}{2}$$

Change $1\frac{1}{2}$ to $\frac{3}{2}$

Change $4\frac{1}{2}$ to $\frac{9}{2}$

Multiply $\frac{3}{2} \times \frac{9}{2} = \frac{27}{4}$ or $6\frac{3}{4}$

$$Answer = 6\frac{3}{4}$$

Division of Fractions

Dividing a Fraction by Another Fraction

Sometimes it is necessary to divide fractions in order to calculate a drug dosage.

■ **Rule: To Divide Fractions Follow These Steps:**

- Write your problem.

  EXAMPLE: $\dfrac{4}{5} \div \dfrac{5}{9}$

- Invert the number by which you are dividing. This means that 5/9 becomes 9/5.
- Multiply your fractions to get your answer. If you use the example above, your problem now looks like this:

$$\dfrac{4}{5} \times \dfrac{9}{5} = \dfrac{36}{25} = 1\dfrac{11}{25}$$

Answer $= 1\dfrac{11}{25}$

EXAMPLE: $\dfrac{7}{8} \div \dfrac{3}{5}$

Invert $\dfrac{3}{5}$ to $\dfrac{5}{3}$

Multiply $\dfrac{7}{8} \times \dfrac{5}{3} = \dfrac{35}{24} = 1\dfrac{11}{24}$

Answer $= 1\dfrac{11}{24}$

Dividing a Fraction by a Mixed Number

Whenever you have to divide a mixed number, you should always convert the mixed number to an improper fraction before you work your problem.

■ RULE: **To Divide a Fraction That Involves a Mixed Number, Change the Mixed Number to an Improper Fraction.**

EXAMPLE: $\dfrac{3}{6} \div 1\dfrac{2}{5}$

Change $1\dfrac{2}{5}$ to $\dfrac{7}{5}$

Write $\dfrac{3}{6} \div \dfrac{7}{5}$

Invert $\dfrac{7}{5}$ to $\dfrac{5}{7}$

Multiply $\dfrac{3}{6} \times \dfrac{5}{7} = \dfrac{15}{42} = \dfrac{5}{14}$

Answer $= \dfrac{5}{14}$

Practice Problems

Multiplication of Fractions

1. $\dfrac{7}{15} \times \dfrac{8}{12}$

Answer =

2. $\frac{5}{9} \times \frac{3}{7}$

Answer =

3. $\frac{6}{16} \times \frac{2}{5}$

Answer =

4. $2\frac{7}{10} \times \frac{1}{2}$

Answer =

5. $3\frac{4}{8} \times \frac{3}{16}$

Answer =

Division of Fractions

6. $\frac{3}{4} \div \frac{1}{9}$

Answer =

7. $\frac{6}{13} \div \frac{2}{5}$

Answer =

8. $\frac{8}{12} \div \frac{3}{7}$

Answer =

9. $12 \div \frac{1}{3}$

Answer =

10. $8\frac{7}{10} \div 15$

Answer =

End of Chapter Review

Change the unlike fractions to like fractions by finding a common denominator.

1. $\frac{2}{5}, \frac{3}{7}$

Answer =

2. $\frac{7}{5}, \frac{4}{20}$

Answer =

Reduce the following fractions to their lowest terms:

3. $\frac{27}{162}$

Answer =

4. $\frac{16}{128}$

Answer =

Change the following improper fractions to mixed numbers:

5. $\frac{26}{4}$

Answer =

6. $\frac{105}{8}$

Answer =

Change the following mixed numbers to improper fractions:

7. $4\frac{6}{11}$

Answer =

8. $9\frac{2}{23}$

Answer =

Reduce the following fractions to their lowest terms:

9. $\frac{20}{64}$

Answer =

10. $\frac{16}{128}$

Answer =

11. $\frac{7}{63}$

Answer =

Add the following fractions:

12. $\dfrac{1}{9} + \dfrac{7}{9}$

Answer =

13. $\dfrac{5}{6} + \dfrac{3}{6}$

Answer =

14. $\dfrac{1}{9} + \dfrac{3}{4}$

Answer =

15. $6\dfrac{5}{6} + \dfrac{3}{8}$

Answer =

Subtract the following fractions:

16. $\dfrac{5}{12} - \dfrac{3}{12}$

Answer =

17. $\frac{7}{9} - \frac{2}{9}$

Answer =

18. $\frac{3}{4} - \frac{1}{6}$

Answer =

19. $4\frac{6}{10} - \frac{3}{8}$

Answer =

20. $6\frac{3}{8} - 4\frac{1}{4}$

Answer =

Multiply the following fractions:

21. $\frac{6}{8} \times \frac{1}{5}$

Answer =

22. $\dfrac{9}{11} \times \dfrac{1}{3}$

Answer =

23. $2\dfrac{1}{10} \times 6\dfrac{6}{9}$

Answer =

24. $2\dfrac{2}{7} \times 3\dfrac{4}{8}$

Answer =

25. $1\dfrac{5}{11} \times \dfrac{3}{8}$

Answer =

Divide the following fractions:

26. $\dfrac{3}{5} \div \dfrac{7}{20}$

Answer =

27. $\dfrac{8}{9} \div \dfrac{1}{27}$

Answer =

28. $6\dfrac{5}{12} \div \dfrac{15}{24}$

Answer =

29. $7\dfrac{2}{14} \div 80$

Answer =

30. $16 \div \dfrac{32}{160}$

Answer =

Chapter 3

Decimals

Medications are frequently prescribed in decimals, and you will find that many of your dosage problems will be worked out using the decimal format. A decimal indicates the "tenths" of a number. A decimal's value is determined by its position to the right of a decimal point. In other words:

0.2 is read as 2 tenths because the number 2 is one position to the right of the decimal point.

0.03 is read as 3 hundredths because the number 3 is two positions to the right of the decimal point.

0.004 is read as 4 thousandths because the number 4 is three positions to the right of the decimal point.

Figure 3-1 may help you understand a decimal's position.

When reading a decimal, it is important to remember that numbers to the right of the decimal point have a value *less than 1*, and numbers to the left of the decimal point have a value *greater than 1*. Remember the following rule:

■ RULE: **Numbers to the Right of the Decimal Point Have a Value Less Than 1,**

Whole numbers	⬆
Ten thousands	10,000
Thousands	1,000
Hundreds	100
Tens	10
Ones	1
Decimal point	•
Tenths	.1
Hundredths	.01
Thousandths	.001
Ten-thousandths	.0001
Hundred thousandths	.00001
Decimal numbers	⬇

Figure 3–1. Numbers read according to their decimal place value.

and Numbers to the Left of the Decimal Point Have a Value Greater Than 1.

To read a decimal fraction, follow these steps:

■ Read the whole numbers to the left of the decimal point.

- Read the decimal point as "and" or "point."
- Read the decimal number to the right of the decimal point.

EXAMPLES: $\boxed{5}$. $\boxed{2}$ $\boxed{6}$. $\boxed{0\ 3}$ $\boxed{0\ .\ 0\ 0\ 4}$

Read:

|five|and|two tenths|six|and|three hundredths|four thousandths|

Practice Problems

Write the following decimals as you would read them.

1. 10.001

Answer =

2. 3.0007

Answer =

3. 0.083

Answer =

4. 0.153

Answer =

5. 36.0067

Answer =

6. 0.0125

Answer =

7. 125.025

Answer =

8. 20.075

Answer =

Write the following decimals:

9. Five and thirty-seven thousandths

Answer =

10. Sixty-four and seven hundredths

Answer =

11. Twenty thousandths

Answer =

12. Four tenths

Answer =

13. Eight and sixty-four thousandths

Answer =

14. Thirty-three and seven tenths

Answer =

15. Fifteen thousandths

Answer =

16. One tenth

Answer =

Addition of Decimals

■ Rule: **To Add Decimals,
Follow These Steps:**

- Place the decimals to be added in a vertical column with the decimal points directly under one another. If you want to add 0.5, 3.24, and 8.0, then you would place the numbers like this:

$$
\begin{array}{r}
0.50 \\
3.24 \\
+\,8.00 \\
\end{array}
$$

- Add the decimals in the same manner as whole numbers are added:

$$
\begin{array}{r}
0.50 \\
3.24 \\
+\,8.00 \\
\hline
11.74 \\
\end{array}
$$

- Place the decimal in the answer directly under aligned decimal points.
- Add zeros to balance the columns if necessary.

EXAMPLES: $3.9 + 4.7$

$$
\begin{array}{r}
3.9 \\
+\,4.7 \\
\hline
8.6 \\
\end{array}
$$

Answer = 8.6

$$6 + 2.8 + 1.6$$

$$\begin{array}{r} 6.0 \\ 2.8 \\ +\ \ 1.6 \\ \hline 10.4 \end{array}$$

Answer = 10.4

Subtraction of Decimals

■ **RULE: To Subtract Decimals, Follow These Steps:**

- Place the decimals to be subtracted in a vertical column with the decimal points directly under one another. If you want to subtract 4.1 from 6.2, you would place the numbers like this:

$$\begin{array}{r} 6.2 \\ -4.1 \end{array}$$

- Subtract the decimals in the same manner as whole numbers are subtracted.

$$\begin{array}{r} 6.2 \\ -4.1 \\ \hline 2.1 \end{array}$$

- Place the decimal point in the answer directly under the aligned decimal points.
- Add zeros to balance the columns as necessary.

EXAMPLES:

$16.84 - 1.32$

$$\begin{array}{r} 16.84 \\ -\ 1.32 \\ \hline 15.52 \end{array}$$

Answer $= 15.52$

$13.60 - 8.00$

$$\begin{array}{r} 13.60 \\ -\ 8.00 \\ \hline 5.60 \end{array}$$

Answer $= 5.60$

$7.02 - 3.0086$

$$\begin{array}{r} 7.0200 \\ -3.0086 \\ \hline 4.0114 \end{array}$$

Answer $= 4.0114$

Multiplication of Decimals

Multiplication of Decimal Numbers

Multiplication of decimals is done using the same method as is used for multiplying whole numbers. The major concern is placement of the decimal point in the product.

■ **RULE: To Multiply Decimals, Follow These Steps:**

- Place the decimals to be multiplied in the same position as whole numbers would be placed. If you want to multiply 6.3 by 7.6, then place the numbers like this:

$$\begin{array}{r} 6.3 \\ \times 7.6 \\ \hline \end{array}$$

■ Multiply the decimal numbers and write down the product:

$$
\begin{array}{r}
6.3 \\
\times\,7.6 \\
\hline
378 \\
441 \\
\hline
4788
\end{array}
$$

■ Count off the number of decimal places *to the right* of the decimal in the two numbers being multiplied and count off the total number of places in the product. For example:

  6.3 one place to right of decimal
  × 7.6 + one place to right of decimal
    378
    441
  47.88 two places, count off right to left
    ↑

Answer = 47.88

Multiplication by 10, 100, or 1000

Multiplying by 10, 100 or 1000 is a fast and easy way to calculate dosage problems. Simply move the decimal point the same number of places to the right as there are zeros in the multiplier. See Table 3–1.

EXAMPLES: 0.712 × 10. There is one zero in the multiplier of ten. Move the decimal one place to the right for an answer of 7.12.

Table 3-1. Multiplying by 10, 100, or 1000		
MULTIPLIER	NUMBER OF ZEROS	MOVE THE DECIMAL
10	1	1 place
100	2	2 places
1000	3	3 places

0.08×1000. There are three zeros in the multiplier of 1000. Move the decimal three places to the right for an answer of 80.

Division of Decimals

Division of Decimal Numbers

Division of decimals is done using the same method as is used for division of whole numbers. The special concern is movement and placement of the decimal point in the divisor, dividend, and quotient.

$$\overset{\text{Quotient}}{\text{Divisor)}\overline{\text{Dividend}}} \quad \frac{\text{Dividend}}{\text{Divisor}} = \text{Quotient}$$

$$\overset{8}{8)\overline{64}} \quad \frac{64}{8} = 8$$

There will be few instances where you will be dividing decimals to calculate dosage problems. When you have to divide decimals, the most important thing to remember is placement of the decimal in the quotient. Review this helpful rule.

■ **Rule: To Divide a Decimal by a Whole Number, Place the Decimal Point in the Quotient Directly Above the Decimal Point in the Dividend.**

Example: $25.5 \div 5$

$$
\begin{array}{r}
5.1 \\
5\overline{)25.5} \\
25 \\
\hline
5 \\
5 \\
\hline
\end{array}
$$

Answer = 5.1

■ **Rule: To Divide a Decimal by a Decimal, Follow These Steps:**

■ Make the decimal number in the divisor a whole number *first*. If you want to divide 0.32 by 1.6 you would make 1.6 a whole number, 16, by moving the decimal point 1 place to the right.
■ Move the decimal point in the dividend (0.32) the same number of places (1) that you moved the decimal point in the divisor.
■ Divide 3.2 by 16.
■ Place the decimal point in the quotient directly above the decimal point in the dividend.

$$
\begin{array}{r}
.2 \\
16\overline{)3.2} \\
3.2 \\
\end{array}
$$

Answer = 0.2

| Table 3–2. Dividing by 10, 100, or 1000 | | |
DIVISOR	NUMBER OF ZEROS	MOVE THE DECIMAL
10	1	1 place
100	2	2 places
1000	3	3 places

Division by 10, 100, 1000

Dividing by 10, 100, or 1000 is fast and easy. Just move the decimal point the same number of places to the left as there are zeros in the divisor. See Table 3–2.

EXAMPLE: 0.09 ÷ 10. Move the decimal one place to the left for an answer of 0.009.

Practice Problems

Add the following decimals:

1. 16.4 + 21.8

Answer =

2. 0.009 + 18.4

Answer =

3. $67.541 + 17.1$

Answer =

Subtract the following decimals:

4. $366.18 - 122.6$

Answer =

5. $107.16 - 56.1$

Answer =

6. $16.19 - 3.86$

Answer =

Multiply the following decimals:

7. 1.86×12.1

Answer =

8. 0.89×7.65

Answer =

9. 13.001×7.8

Answer =

10. 10.65×100

Answer =

Divide the following decimals:

11. $63.8 \div 0.9$

Answer =

12. $39.7 \div 1.3$

Answer =

13. $98.4 \div 1000$

Answer =

14. $.008 \div 10$

Answer =

Changing Fractions to Decimals

Some fractions may divide evenly when converted into decimals. For example, the fraction 1/4 converts into 0.25 and 1/2 converts into 0.50. If a numerator does not divide evenly into the denominator, then work the division to three places.

$$\frac{1}{6} = \frac{\text{numerator}}{\text{denominator}} \xrightarrow[\text{becomes}]{} \frac{\text{dividend}}{\text{divisor}} = \frac{1}{6} \; 6\overline{)1}$$

■ **RULE: To Convert a Fraction to a Decimal, Divide the Numerator by the Denominator. Follow These Steps:**

- Rewrite the fraction in the division format as shown above; reduce if necessary. $6\overline{)1}$
- Place a decimal point after the whole number in the dividend.
- Add zeros as needed. $6\overline{)1.0}$
- Place the decimal point in the quotient directly above the decimal point in the dividend.

  $6\overline{)1.0}^{\;.}$

- Divide.

EXAMPLES:
$$\frac{1}{8} = 1 \div 8 = 8\overline{)1}$$

$$\begin{array}{r} .125 \\ 8\overline{)1.000} \\ \underline{8} \\ 20 \\ \underline{16} \\ 40 \\ \underline{40} \end{array}$$

Answer = 0.125

$$\frac{5}{20} = \frac{1}{4} = 1 \div 4 = 4\overline{)1} \quad 4\overline{)\begin{array}{r} .25 \\ 1.00 \\ \underline{8} \\ 20 \\ \underline{20} \end{array}}$$

Answer = 0.25

$$\frac{6}{30} = \frac{1}{5} = 1 \div 5 = 5\overline{)1} \quad 5\overline{)\begin{array}{r} .2 \\ 1.0 \\ \underline{1\ 0} \end{array}}$$

Answer = 0.2

Changing Decimals to Fractions

When changing decimals to fractions, the decimal number expressed becomes the numerator of the fractions. For example, $0.75 = \frac{75}{?}$. The decimal number places to the right of the decimal will tell you what the denominator is. For example:

> 1 place = a denominator of 10
>
> 2 places = a denominator of 100
>
> 3 places = a denominator of 1000

Therefore, 0.75 is expressed as 75/100.

■ **RULE: To Change a Decimal to a Fraction, Follow These Steps:**

- The decimal number becomes the numerator.

- The number of places to the right of the decimal point determines the denominator's value.
- Write the decimal fraction and reduce if necessary.

EXAMPLES: 0.5   The number 5 becomes the numerator.

$$\frac{5}{?}$$

There is one place to the right of the decimal, which equals a denominator of 10.

The fraction becomes $\frac{5}{10} = \frac{1}{2}$

Rounding Off Decimals

Most decimals are "rounded off" to the hundredth place to ensure accuracy of calculations. Because this process is infrequently done in the clinical setting, it is explained in Appendix A for those of you who wish to review the steps.

Practice Problems

Convert the following fractions to decimals:

1. $\frac{6}{30}$

Answer =

2. $\frac{8}{64}$

Answer =

3. $\frac{15}{60}$

Answer =

4. $\frac{12}{180}$

Answer =

5. $\frac{16}{240}$

Answer =

Convert the following decimals to fractions:

6. 0.007

Answer =

7. 0.93

Answer =

8. 0.412

Answer =

9. 5.03

Answer =

10. 12.2

Answer =

End of Chapter Review

Write the following decimals as you would read them:

1. 5.04 *Answer* =

2. 10.65 *Answer* =

3. 0.008 *Answer* =

Write the following decimals:

4. six and eight hundredths

Answer =

5. one hundred twenty-four and three tenths

Answer =

6. sixteen and one thousandths

Answer =

Solve the following decimal problems:

7. 16.35 (+) 8.1

Answer =

8. 0.062 (+) 59.2

Answer =

9. 7.006 − 4.23

Answer =

10. 15.610 − 10.4

Answer =

11. 27.05 × 8.3

Answer =

12. 0.009×14.2

Answer =

13. $18.75 \div 12$

Answer =

14. $1.070 \div 0.20$

Answer =

Convert the following fractions to decimals and decimals to fractions:

15. $\dfrac{6}{10}$

Answer =

16. $\dfrac{8}{20}$

Answer =

17. $\dfrac{12}{84}$

Answer =

18. 0.45

Answer =

19. 6.8

Answer =

20. 0.75

Answer =

Chapter 4

Percent, Ratio, and Proportion

The use of percentages is common to many disciplines and frequently encountered in the medical and nursing professions. Physicians prescribe solutions for external application (soaks, compresses), as well as internal use (gargles, irrigations, intravenous infusions). Nurses find themselves, sometimes daily, working with drugs and solutions prepared in percentage strength.

Today, pharmacists prepare most percentage strength solutions. In fact, many that are used for external application are prepackaged by pharmaceutical companies. However, some institutions and home health care settings still require the preparation of solutions by nurses, and this will be covered in Chapter 15. This chapter will focus on the basic mathematical skills necessary to calculate percentage problems and will provide the foundation for understanding the preparation of solutions.

Percents

A *percent*

- Refers to the number of units of something compared to the whole.
- Is always a division of 100.

- Is expressed as the "hundredth part."
- Is written with the symbol %, which means "of one hundred."
- Can be written as:
  - A fraction where the denominator is 100.
  - As a decimal by taking the unit to the hundredth part.

The *percent symbol* can be found with:

- A whole number: 20%
- A fraction number: 1/2%
- A mixed number: 20 1/2%
- A decimal number: 20.5%

Fractions and Percents

Sometimes it will be necessary for you to change a percent to a fraction or a fraction to a percent to make dosage calculations easier.

Changing a Percent to a Fraction

▪ **RULE: To Change a Percent to a Fraction, Follow These Steps:**

- Drop the % symbol. 20% →20
- Divide the number by 100. 20 ÷ 100 = 1/5
- Reduce the fraction to its lowest terms.
- Change to a mixed number if necessary.

EXAMPLE: 40%

Change: $40\% = 40 = \dfrac{40}{100}$

Reduce:
$$\frac{40}{100} = \frac{2}{5}$$

$$Answer = \frac{2}{5}$$

EXAMPLE:
$$\frac{1}{2}\%$$

Change:
$$\frac{1}{2}\% = \frac{1}{2} = \frac{\frac{1}{2}}{100}$$

$$\frac{1}{2} \div 100 = \frac{1}{2} \times \frac{1}{100} = \frac{1}{200}$$

$$Answer = \frac{1}{200}$$

Changing a Fraction to a Percent

■ **RULE: To Change a Fraction to a Percent, Follow These Steps:**

- Multiply the fraction by 100. For 1/2, multiply $1/2 \times 100 = 100/2$.
- Reduce if necessary. $100/2 = 50$
- Change any improper fraction to a mixed number.
- Add % symbol. 50%

EXAMPLE:
$$\frac{3}{4}$$

Change:
$$\frac{3}{\underset{1}{4}} \times \overset{25}{100} = \frac{75}{1} = 75$$

Add % symbol. 75%

Answer = 75%

EXAMPLE: $\dfrac{3}{5}$

Change: $\dfrac{3}{5} \times 100 = \dfrac{3}{\cancel{5}_1} \times \dfrac{\cancel{100}^{20}}{1} = 60$

Add % symbol. 60%

Answer = 60%

EXAMPLE: $6\dfrac{1}{2}$

Change: $6\dfrac{1}{2} \times 100$

Change $6\dfrac{1}{2}$ to an improper fraction.

$6\dfrac{1}{2} = \dfrac{13}{2}$

$\dfrac{13}{2} \times 100 = \dfrac{13}{\cancel{2}_1} \times \dfrac{\cancel{100}^{50}}{1} = 650$

Add % symbol. 650%

Answer = 650%

Practice Problems

Change the following percents to fractions:

1. 15% = _____

2. 30% = _____

3. 50% = _____

4. 75% = _____

5. 25% = _____

6. 60% = _____

Change the following fractions to percents:

7. $\frac{1}{3}$ = _____

8. $\frac{2}{3}$ = _____

9. $\frac{1}{5}$ = _____

10. $\frac{3}{4}$ = _____

11. $\frac{2}{5}$ = _____

12. $\frac{1}{4}$ = _____

Decimals and Percents

Sometimes it will be necessary for you to change a percent to a decimal or a decimal to a percent to make dosage calculations easier.

Changing a Percent to a Decimal

■ RULE: **To Change a Percent to a Decimal, Follow These Steps:**

- Drop the % symbol. When you drop a % symbol from a whole number, a decimal point takes the place of the symbol. For example, when you drop the % symbol from 68%, the decimal point replaces the % symbol (68.0).
- Divide by 100 by moving the decimal point two places to the left. 68.0 = 68. = 0.68
- Add zeros as needed.

EXAMPLE: 36%

Change: $36\% = 36\% = 36.$ } decimal replaces % symbol

$36. = .36. = 0.36$ } move the decimal point to the left

Answer = 0.36

EXAMPLE: 14.1%

Change: $14.1\% = 14.1\% = 14.1$

$14.1 = .14.1 = 0.141$

Answer = 0.141

Changing a Decimal to a Percent

■ RULE: **To Change a Decimal to a Percent, Follow These Steps:**

- Multiply by 100 by moving the decimal point two places to the right. For 3.19 you would move the decimal point two places to the right, so 3.19 = 3.19 = 319
- Add zeros as needed.
- Add the % symbol. 319 = 319%

EXAMPLE: 1.61

Change: $1.61 \times 100 = 1.61 = 161$
                $161 = 161\%$

Answer = 161%

EXAMPLE: 0.032

Change: $0.032 \times 100 = 0.03.2 = 3.2$
                $3.2 = 3.2\%$

Answer = 3.2%

Practice Problems

Change the following percents to a decimal:

1. 15% = _____

2. 25% = _____

3. 50% = _____

4. 80% = _____

Change the following decimals to percents:

5. 0.25 = _____

6. 0.45 = _____

7. 0.60 = _____

8. 0.85 = _____

Ratio and Proportion

A *ratio* is used to express a relationship between two units or quantities by division. A slash (/) or colon (:) is used to indicate division, and both are read as "is to" or "per." For the ratio of 1 is to 2, you can write 1:2 or 1/2. The *numerator* is *always to the left* of the colon or slash and the *denominator is always to the right* of the colon or slash.

A *proportion* states that two ratios are equal. A proportion can be written in a fraction form in which the numerator and denominator of one fraction have the same relationship as the numerator and denominator of another fraction. The equal symbol (=) is read as "as." For example:

$$\left.\frac{1}{3} = \frac{3}{9}\right\} \text{ 1 is to 3 } as \text{ 3 is to 9}$$

A proportion can also be written in a colon format in which the ratio to the left of the double colon is equal to the ratio to the right of the double colon. The double colon (::) is read as "as." For example:

1:3 :: 3:9} 1 is to 3 *as* 3 is to 9

In this example, the first and fourth terms are called *extremes,* while the second and third terms are called the *means*.

$$\overbrace{1{:}3 :: 3{:}9}^{\text{EXTREMES}}$$

MEANS

■ RULE: **In a Proportion, the Product of the Extremes is Always Equal to the Product of the Means.**

To verify that two ratios in a proportion are equal:

■ *For a fraction,* multiply the numerator of each ratio by its opposite denominator.

Sum products will be equal.

EXAMPLE: $\dfrac{1}{3} : \dfrac{3}{9}$

$\dfrac{1}{3} \diagdown : \diagup \dfrac{3}{9}$

$$1 \times 9 = 9$$
$$3 \times 3 = 9$$
$$9 = 9$$

- *For a ratio*, multiply the extremes and then multiply the means.

The product of the means equals the product of the extremes.

EXAMPLES: 1:3 :: 3:9

1:3 :: 3:9

$$1 \times 9 = 9$$
$$3 \times 3 = 9$$
$$9 = 9$$

Practice Problems

Write the following relationships in ratio form, using both the fraction and colon format:

1. Amoxil pediatric drops contain 50 milligrams of amoxicillin in 5 milliliters of solution.

2. There are 325 milligrams of acetaminophen in 1 tablet of Tylenol.

3. Each liter of dextrose solution contains 2 ampules of multivitamins.

Write the following relationships as a proportion, using both the fraction and colon format:

4. Each aspirin tablet contains 5 grains of ace-tylsalicylic acid (ASA). The nurse is to give 3 aspirin tablets equal to 15 grains of ASA.

5. Catapres is available in 0.2 milligram tablets. A patient was prescribed 0.4 milligrams/day provided by 2 tablets.

6. Alupent is available in syrup form as 10 milli-grams/5 milliliters. A patient is to take 30 milli-grams or 15 milliliters during a 24-hour period.

Solving for x

Frequently in dosage calculation problems it is nec-essary to find an unknown quantity. In a proportion problem, the unknown quantity is identified as x. Read the following word problem and solve for x.

EXAMPLE: Demerol 75 milligrams is prescribed for postoperative pain. The medication is available as 100 milligrams in 1 mil-liliter. To administer the prescribed dose of 75 milligrams, the nurse would give _____ milliliter(s).

■ RULE: To Solve for x Using a Fraction Format, Follow the Steps Below:

- Write down what is available or *what you have* in a fraction format. For this example, you should write:

$$\frac{100 \text{ mg}}{1 \text{ ml}}$$

- Complete the proportion by writing down what you desire in a fraction format, making sure that the numerators are like units and the denominators are like units:

$$\frac{100 \text{ mg}}{1 \text{ ml}} :: \frac{75 \text{ mg}}{x \text{ ml}}$$

- Cross multiply the numerator of each ratio by its opposite denominator:

$$\frac{100 \text{ mg}}{1 \text{ ml}} \diagdown :: \diagup \frac{75 \text{ mg}}{x \text{ ml}}$$

By doing this you should get the following proportion:

$$100 \text{ mg} \times x \text{ ml} = 75 \text{ mg} \times 1 \text{ ml}$$
$$100x = 75$$

- Solve for x by dividing both sides of the equation by the number before x. In this case, the number before x is 100, so divide both sides of the equation by 100:

$$\frac{100x}{100} = \frac{75}{100}$$

$$\frac{\cancel{100}x}{\cancel{100}} = \frac{75}{100}$$

$$x = \frac{3}{4}\text{ml}$$

$$Answer = \frac{3}{4} \text{ ml}$$

■ **RULE: To Solve for *x* Using a Colon Format, Follow These Steps:**

EXAMPLE: Demerol 75 milligrams is prescribed for postoperative pain. The medication is available as 100 milligrams in 1 milliliter. To administer the prescribed dose of 75 milligrams, the nurse would have to give _____ milliliter(s).

■ Write down what is available or *what you have* in a colon format. For this example, you should write:

$$100 \text{ mg} : 1 \text{ ml}$$

■ Complete the proportion by writing down *what you desire,* making sure that the numerators are like units and the denominators are like units.

$$100 \text{ mg} : 1 \text{ ml} :: 75 \text{ mg} : x \text{ ml}$$

■ Multiply the extremes:

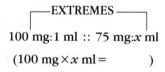

$$100 \text{ mg} : 1 \text{ ml} :: 75 \text{ mg} : x \text{ ml}$$

$$(100 \text{ mg} \times x \text{ ml} = \qquad)$$

■ Multiply the means:

$$100 \text{ mg}:1 \text{ ml} :: 75 \text{ mg}:x \text{ ml}$$
$$\underset{\text{MEANS}}{\lfloor\qquad\qquad\rfloor}$$

$$(\qquad = 75 \text{ mg} \times 1 \text{ ml})$$

■ Complete the equation $100 \text{ mg} \times x \text{ ml} = 75 \text{ mg} \times 1 \text{ ml}$:

$$100x = 75$$

■ Solve for x. (Remember: divide both sides of the equation by the number before x [100].)

$$\frac{100x}{100} = \frac{75}{100}$$
$$\frac{\cancel{100}x}{\cancel{100}} = \frac{75}{100}$$
$$x = \frac{3}{4}\text{ml}$$

$$\textit{Answer} = \frac{3}{4} \text{ ml}$$

■ Verify the accuracy of the answer, $x = 3/4$ ml.
■ For the fraction format, multiply the numerator of each ratio by its opposite denominator. The sum products will be equal.

$$\frac{100 \text{ mg}}{1 \text{ ml}} : \frac{75 \text{ mg}}{\frac{3}{4} \text{ ml}}$$

$$\overset{25}{\cancel{100}} \times \frac{3}{\cancel{4}} = 75 \left.\begin{array}{l} \\ \\ \\ \\ \end{array}\right\} \begin{array}{l} \text{Sum} \\ \text{products} \\ \text{are} \\ \text{equal} \end{array}$$

$$1 \times 75 = 75$$

- For the colon format, multiply the means, then multiply the extremes. The product of the means will equal the product of the extremes.

$$\overset{\overbrace{\hspace{3.2cm}}^{\text{EXTREMES}}}{100 \text{ mg} : 1 \text{ ml} :: 75 \text{ mg} : \frac{3}{4} \text{ ml}}$$
$$\underbrace{\hspace{2.5cm}}_{\text{MEANS}}$$

$$75 \times 1 = 75$$
$$100 \times \frac{3}{4} = \frac{\overset{25}{\cancel{100}}}{1} \times \frac{3}{\cancel{4}} = 75 \left.\begin{array}{l} \\ \\ \\ \\ \end{array}\right\} \begin{array}{l} \text{Sum} \\ \text{products} \\ \text{are} \\ \text{equal} \end{array}$$

Practice Problems

1. The physician prescribed 1 milligram of folic acid, by injection, once per day. The medication is available as 5 mg/ml. The nurse would give _____ ml.

2. Apresoline 30 milligrams was prescribed three times a day. The medication is available as 10 milligram tablets. The nurse would give _____ tablet(s) three times per day.

3. Aldomet 250 milligrams was prescribed every 6 hours. The drug is available in 125 mg tablets. The nurse would give _____ tablet(s) every 6 hours.

End of Chapter Review

Change the following:

Percent	*Fraction*	*Decimal*
1. _____	1/6	_____
2. _____	_____	0.25
3. 6.4%	_____	_____
4. 21%	_____	_____
5. _____	2/5	_____
6. _____	_____	1.62
7. _____	_____	0.27
8. 5 2/8%	_____	_____
9. _____	9/2	_____
10. 8 3/9%	_____	_____
11. 31%	_____	_____

12. _____   6/7   _____

13. _____   18/4   _____

14. _____   _____   1.5

15. _____   _____   0.72

Write the following ratios in fraction and colon format:

16. Chewable Cardilate tablets contain 10 milligrams of erythrityl tetranitrate in each tablet.

    _____ fraction   _____ colon

17. Pitocin is available for injection as 10 units in each milliliter.

    _____ fraction   _____ colon

18. For a serious infection a physician could prescribe 200 milligrams of Azlocillin for every kilogram of body weight.

    _____ fraction   _____ colon

19. The physician ordered 300 milligrams of quinidine sulfate. The tablets were available in 100 milligrams per tablet.

    _____ fraction   _____ ratio

20. Dymelor 500 milligrams was ordered for a patient every morning. The medication was

available in 250 milligram tablets.

_____ fraction   _____ ratio

21. Synthroid is available in 0.075 milligram tablets. A physician ordered 0.15 milligrams
daily.

_____ fraction   _____ ratio

Solve for x for the remaining problems and verify
your answer using a fraction or colon format.

22. The physician prescribed 10 milligrams of
Vasoxyl for moderate postoperative hypoten-
sion. The medication was available as 20 milligrams in 1 milliliter. The nurse would give
_____ milliliter(s).

Verify your answer:

23. The physician prescribed 25 milligrams of meperidine hydrochloride syrup to be given every 3 hours for pain as needed. The syrup preparation was available as 50 milligrams in 5 milliliters. To give 25 milligrams the nurse would give _____ milliliter(s).

Verify your answer:

24. The physician ordered 1.5 milligrams of leucovorin calcium for nutritional deficiency. The medication was available as 3.0 milligrams in a 1.0 milliliter ampule. The nurse would give _____ milliliter(s).

Verify your answer:

Unit II

Measurement Systems

The metric and apothecaries' systems of weights and measures are in wide use today as they have been for many years. While the apothecaries' system is still used today by many health care practitioners, with the current shift in health delivery from the institution to the home, the use of household measurements is becoming more popular.

To effectively deliver medications today, nurses need to be familiar with all three systems of measurement and to become expert at converting from one unit of measure to another, within the same system, or between two systems. This unit will present the metric and apothecaries' systems as well as household measurements. The reader will be shown "how to" convert among all measurements. Equivalent values have been listed to facilitate conversions and dosage calculations.

Chapter 5

The Metric System

The metric system is a decimal system based on multiples of ten. Portions can be increased or decreased by multiples of ten (10, 100, 1000). This can be achieved by moving the decimal point to the right for multiplication or to the left for division.

$$1.0 \ \textit{increased by} \ 10 = 1.\underset{\uparrow}{0} = 10$$

$$0.1 \ \textit{decreased by} \ 10 = \underset{\uparrow}{0}.1 = 0.01$$

The metric system has three basic units of measurement: length (meter), volume (liter), and weight (gram).

Meter—Length

A meter is:

- The basic unit of length
- Equal to 39.37 inches
- Abbreviated as m or M

The primary linear measurements used in medicine are centimeters and millimeters. Centimeters are used for measuring such things as the size of body organs and wounds; millimeters are used for blood pressure measurements. The important units of metric length can be found in Table 5–1.

You can move about from point to point on the above system.

■ Rule: **To Move from Smaller to Larger, Follow These Steps:**

- Count the number of places to be moved.
- Move the decimal point *to the left* the number of places counted.

Example: Change millimeter (6000) to decimeter:
Count two places to be moved.
Move two places to the left.

60 00.   60

(milli) = (deci)

Answer = 60

■ Rule: **To Move from Larger to Smaller, Follow These Steps:**

- Count the number of places to be moved.
- Move the decimal point *to the right* the number of places counted.

Table 5–1. Units of Metric Length		
1 meter =	10 decimeters (dm)	
	100 centimeters (cm)	
	1000 millimeters (mm)	

EXAMPLE: Change deci (80) to centi.
            Count one place to be moved.
            Move one place to the right.

    80.   800
    └┘
    (deci) = (centi)

                                    Answer = 800

Practice Problems

Change the following units of metric length:

1. 3.60 cm = _____ M

2. 4.16 M = _____ dm

3. 0.8 mm = _____ cm

4. 2 mm = _____ M

Liter—Volume

A liter is:

- A basic unit of volume.
- The total amount of water in a cube that measures 10 cm × 10 cm × 10 cm (= cm³).
- A cube 10 cm³ (see Figure 5–1).
- Equal to 1000 ml = 1000 cc.
- Abbreviated as 1 or L.

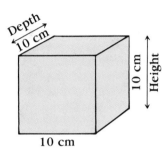

Figure 5-1. Cube measuring 10 cm on all sides = 1 liter.

It is important to note that 1 liter equals 1000 ml, which also equals 1000 cc. The units of metric volume can be found in Table 5–2.

The rules for moving from larger to smaller and from smaller to larger that you used for units of metric length can also be used for units of metric volume and weight.

Gram—Weight

A gram is:

- A basic unit of weight.
- The weight of distilled water in 1 cubic centimeter at a temperature of 4 degrees centigrade.

Table 5-2. Units of Metric Volume	
1 liter =	10 deciliters (dl)
	100 centiliters (cl)
	1000 milliliters (ml)

- A cube 1.0 cm^3 (see Figure 5-2).
- Equal to a volume of 1 ml in 1 cc.
- Abbreviated as g.

The units of metric weight can be found in Table 5-3.

Practice Problems

Change the following units of metric volume and weight.

1. 3.006 ml = _____ L

2. 6.17 cl = _____ ml

3. 0.9 L = _____ ml

4. 6.40 cg = _____ mg

5. 1000 mg = _____ g

6. 0.8 mg = _____ dg

End of Chapter Review

Change the following units of metric length:

1. 7.43 mm = _____ M

2. 0.06 cm = _____ dm

3. 10 Km = _____ M

4. 62.17 dm = _____ mm

Change the following units of metric volume:

5. 1.64 ml = _____ dl

6. 0.47 dl = _____ L

7. 10 L = _____ cl

8. 56.9 cl = _____ ml

Change the following units of metric weight:

9. 35.6 mg = _____ g

10. 0.3 g = _____ cg

11. 0.05 g = _____ mg

12. 93 cg = _____ mg

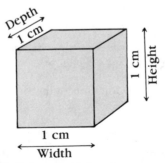

Figure 5–2. Cube measuring 1 cm on all sides = 1 gram.

Table 5-3. Units of Metric Weight

$$1 \text{ gram} = \begin{cases} 10 \text{ decigrams (dg)} \\ 100 \text{ centigrams (cg)} \\ 1000 \text{ milligrams (mg)} \end{cases}$$

1 milligram = 1000 micrograms (μg or mcg)
1 kilogram = 1000 grams

13. 100 mcg = _____ mg

14. 2 mg = _____ mcg

15. 1.0 mcg = _____ mg

Chapter 6

The Apothecaries' System

The apothecaries' system of measurement, while less popular today than the metric system, is still used by physicians, especially for prescribing medications that have been used for many years (*e.g.,* digitalis, aspirin).

Documentation in the apothecaries' system requires *writing the symbol before the quantity.* The quantity should be recorded in Roman numerals;* for example, 6 fluidrams should be written as f℥vi. Arabic numerals can be used for large quantities or when the amount is to be written out; *i.e.,* 10 drams, 9 fluidounces. Arabic numerals are also used to express fractional quantities (1/2, 1/4, 1/50) although ss or s̈s is an acceptable symbol for 1/2.

The apothecaries' system has two basic units of measurement:

Unit	Term	
Weight	Grain	
Volume	Minim	= Drop

A grain is equal to the weight of a grain of wheat; the minim is equal to the quantity of water in a drop that also weighs 1 grain.

---

*Refer to Chapter 1 to review Roman numerals.

Table 6-1. Apothecary Units of Weight

UNIT	WEIGHT	SYMBOL
Grain*	—	gr
Dram	60 grains	ℨ
Ounce	8 drams	℥ or oz
Pound	12 ounces†	lb

*The grain is the basic unit.
†A pound in this system is equal to 12 ounces; a pound in the English system is equal to 16 ounces.

Table 6-2. Apothecary Units of Volume

UNIT	VOLUME	SYMBOL
Minim*	1 drop of water	m
Fluidram†	60 minims	fℨ
Fluidounce†	8 fluidrams	f℥
Pint	16 fluidounces	pt or 0
Quart	2 pints	qt
Gallon	4 quarts	gal or C

*The minim is the basic unit.
†When the substance is known to be a liquid, the term fluid does not have to be used.

Sometimes it will be necessary to change from one unit to another within the same system.

■ RULE: To Change Units Within the Same System, Follow These Steps:‡

- Look up the equivalent values in the system. For example, if you want to know how many ounces there are in 20 drams then look up the equivalent value of 8 drams = 1 ounce.

‡ Refer to page 81 to review solving for "x."

- Write down *what you know* in a ratio or fraction format:

$$\frac{8 \text{ drams}}{1 \text{ ounce}}$$

- Write down *what you desire* in a ratio or fraction format to complete the proportion. The unknown value is referred to as *x*:

$$\frac{8 \text{ drams}}{1 \text{ ounce}} :: \frac{20 \text{ drams}}{x \text{ ounces}}$$

- Cross multiply to get the following:

$$8 \text{ drams} \times x \text{ ounces} = 20 \text{ drams} \times 1 \text{ ounce}$$
$$8x = 20$$

- Solve for *x* (divide both sides of the equation by the number before the $x = 8$):

$$\frac{8x}{8} = \frac{20}{8}$$

$$\frac{\overset{1}{\cancel{8}}x}{\underset{2}{\cancel{8}}} = \frac{\overset{5}{\cancel{20}}}{\underset{1}{\cancel{8}}}$$

$$x = \frac{5}{2} = 2\frac{1}{2}$$

Answer $= 2\frac{1}{2}$ ounces

End of Chapter Review

Write the following, using Roman numerals and symbols:

1. 3 grains _____

2. 5 drams _____

3. 8 fluidrams _____

4. 10 minims _____

5. 20 1/2 minims _____

6. 5 pints _____

Solve the following:

7. 8 quarts = _____ gallon(s)

8. f ʒ ii = _____ minim(s)

9. f ʒ iv = _____ fluidram(s)

10. grxxx = _____ dram(s)

11. f ʒ viii = _____ ounces(s)

12. 4 pints = _____ quart(s)

Chapter 7

Household Measurements

Household measurements are determined by using containers easily found in the home. Common household measuring devices are those utensils used for cooking, eating, and measuring liquid proportions. They include medicine droppers, teaspoons, tablespoons, cups, and glasses. Because containers differ in design, size, and capacity, it is impossible to establish a standard unit of measure. Probably the *most common* measuring device found in the home is the measuring cup, which calibrates ounces and cups and is available for liquid and dry measures (Figure 7–1). Additionally,

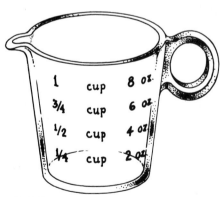

Figure 7–1. Measuring cup (1-cup capacity)—a common household container.

many families have a 1-ounce measuring cup that calibrates teaspoons and/or tablespoons (Figure 7-2). Some pharmaceutical companies package 1-ounce measuring cups or calibrated medicine droppers with their over-the-counter medications (Ny-Quil, Children's Liquid Tylenol). Hospitals commonly use a standard 1-ounce measuring cup (Figure 7-3). The calibrated containers use the metric and apothecaries' systems.

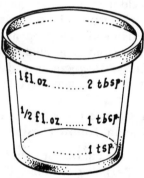

Figure 7-2. One-ounce measuring cup.

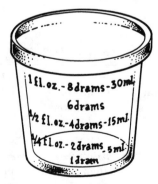

Figure 7-3. One-ounce measuring cup commonly used in hospitals and similar institutions.

Household measurements are approximate in comparison to the exactness of the metric and apothecaries' systems. However, they are frequently used and do have equivalent values in the other systems. For consistency within the system, a drop is equal to a drop, regardless of the liquid's viscosity.

When measuring a liquid medication, it is important that the container/dropper be held so the calibrations are at eye level. When a container/dropper is held at eye level, the liquid will appear to be uneven or U-shaped. This curve, called a *meniscus*, is caused by surface tension; its shape is influenced by the viscosity of the fluid. When measuring the level of a liquid medication, read the calibration "at the bottom" of the meniscus (Figure 7–4).

■ **RULE: To Change Units Within the Same System, Follow These Steps:**

- Look up the equivalent values in the system (Table 7–1). For example, if you want to

Table 7–1. Common Household Quantities

UNIT	VOLUME	SYMBOL
Drop	—	gtt
Teaspoon	60 drops	t or tsp
Tablespoon	3 teaspoons	T or tbsp
Ounce	2 tablespoons	oz
Cup	6 ounces*	c
Glass	8 ounces	—
Pint	16 ounces	pt
Quart	2 pints	qt

*Refers to a teacup, not a measuring cup.

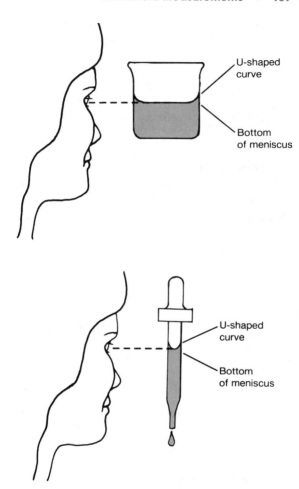

Figure 7–4. Liquid medication being read at the bottom of the meniscus; container or dropper is held at eye level.

know how many ounces there are in 4 table-spoons, then look up the equivalent value of 1 ounce = 2 tablespoons.

■ Write down *what you know* in a fraction or ratio format.

$$\left(\frac{2 \text{ tbs}}{1 \text{ oz}} \text{ or } 2 \text{ tbs}:1 \text{ oz}\right)$$

■ Write down *what you desire* in a fraction or ratio format to complete the proportion. The unknown unit is referred to as x. Consider the fraction format here.

$$\frac{2 \text{ tbs}}{1 \text{ oz}} : \frac{4 \text{ tbs}}{x}$$

■ Cross-multiply to get the following:

$$2 \text{ tbs} \times x \text{ oz} = 4 \text{ tbs} \times 1 \text{ oz}$$
$$2x = 4$$

Solve for x:

$$\frac{2x}{2} = \frac{4}{2}$$

$$\frac{\overset{1}{\cancel{2}x}}{\underset{1}{\cancel{2}}} = \frac{\overset{2}{\cancel{4}}}{\underset{1}{\cancel{2}}}$$

$$x = 2$$

Answer = 2 ounces

Sometimes it is helpful to memorize the equivalent units and quickly convert within the same system.

End of Chapter Review

1. 12 ounces = _____ cup(s)

2. 3 glasses = _____ ounces

3. 6 tablespoons = _____ ounces(s)

4. 2 teaspoons = _____ drops

5. 3 tablespoons = _____ teaspoons

6. 2 cups = _____ ounces

7. 8 ounces = _____ pint

8. 2 glasses = _____ pint

Chapter 8

System Equivalents
and System Conversions

Many times a drug is prescribed in a unit different
from the unit that is available. Previous chapters
(5, 6, and 7) have shown you how to change from
one unit to another *within the same system.* This
chapter will show you how to convert units from
two different systems. To successfully convert between systems, you should memorize certain essential equivalent values among units. It must be
remembered that equivalent values are just that,
equivalent—almost but not quite equal. When re-
cording equivalent values, numerals are rounded
off to facilitate drug calculations.

To make conversions from one system to another easier it is necessary to memorize the following equivalents (Table 8–1).

The metric and English equivalents for length
are rarely used for drug dosage calculations but
can be used when applying a paste, cream, or
ointment that needs to cover a certain area; *e.g.,*
topical nitroglycerin ointment. However, both are
used for linear measurements; *e.g.,* wound size,
head circumference, abdominal girth, and height
(Table 8–2).

Table 8-1. Volume and Weight Equivalents

METRIC SYSTEM	APOTHECARIES' SYSTEM	HOUSEHOLD MEASUREMENTS
Volume		
—	1 minim	1 drop
1 milliliter	15–16 minims	15–16 drops
4–5 milliliters	1 fluidram (60 minims)	1 teaspoon
15 milliliters	4 fluidrams	1 tablespoon (3–4 teaspoons)
30 milliliters	1 fluidounce (8 fluidrams)	2 tablespoons (1 ounce)
180 milliliters	6 ounces	1 cup
240 milliliters	8 ounces	1 glass
500 milliliters	1 pint	—
1000 milliliters (1 liter)	1 quart	—
Weight		
0.60–0.65 milligrams	gr 1/100	—
0.5 milligrams	gr 1/120	—
0.4 milligrams	gr 1/150	—
0.3 milligrams	gr 1/200	—
0.2 milligrams	gr 1/300	—
1000 micrograms	gr 1/60	—
1.0 mg	gr 1/60	—
6.0 mg	gr 1/10	—
60–65 milligrams	1 grain	—
1 gram	15 grains	—
4–5 grams	1 dram	—
30 grams	8 drams	1 ounce
454 grams	—	1 pound
1 kilogram	—	2.2 pounds

Table 8-2. Linear Equivalents
for the English and
Metric Systems

ENGLISH	METRIC
1 inch	2.5 centimeters
12 inches (1 foot)	30 centimeters
39.4 inches (1 yard)	1 meter

System Conversions Using Volume and Weight Units

■ **RULE: To Solve for "*x*" When Converting Between Systems, Follow These Steps:**

■ Look up the equivalent value between the systems. For example, if you wanted to know how many grams there are in 30 grains you would look up the equivalent value of 15 grains = 1 gram.

■ Write down *what you have* in a fraction or colon format:

15 grains:1 gram

■ Complete the proportion by writing down *what you desire:*

15 grains:1 gram::30 grains:*x* grams

■ Multiply the means and the extremes:

$$15x = 30$$

■ Solve for x:

$$\frac{15x}{15} = \frac{30}{15}$$

$$\frac{\overset{1}{\cancel{15x}}}{\underset{1}{\cancel{15}}} = \frac{\overset{2}{\cancel{30}}}{\underset{1}{\cancel{15}}}$$

$$x = 2 \text{ grams}$$

Answer = 2 grams

Practice Problems

Complete the following. Solve for "x" or the unknown by using a fraction or colon format.

1. 12 fluidrams = _____ milliliter(s)

2. 3 milliliters = _____ minim(s)

3. 2 teaspoons = _____ milliliter(s)

Complete the following. Solve for x or the unknown by using a fraction or colon format.

4. gr 1/200 = _____ milligram(s)

5. 6 drams = _____ gram(s)

6. 30 ml = _____ ounce(s)

7. 6 mg = _____ grain(s)

8. 1 liter = _____ quart(s)

9. 2.2 lbs = _____ Kilogram(s)

End of Chapter Review

Complete the following. Solve for x by using a fraction or colon format.

1. A child who weighs 55 pounds weighs _____ kilogram(s).

2. Two (2) ounces of metamucil powder would be equivalent to _____ gram(s).

3. A patient is restricted to four 8-ounce glasses of water per day. The nurse knows that the

patient's fluid intake is restricted to _____ milliliters per day.

4. A patient's abdominal wound measures 10 centimeters in diameter. The nurse knows this is equivalent to _____ inch(es).

5. A child was prescribed 1 fluidram of cough syrup, four times a day, as needed. The child's mother administered _____ teaspoon(s) each time the medication was given.

6. The nurse administered aspirin gr v. She knew this was equivalent to _____ milligram(s).

7. The nurse instilled 3 minims of Lacrisert into the patient's right eye, three times per day. The nurse knew that 3 minims was equal to _____ drop(s).

8. The physician prescribed 0.4 milligrams of atropine sulfate to be administered intramuscularly. The medication was labeled in grains/ml. The nurse knew to look for an ampule labeled _____ grains/ml.

9. A patient was to take 2 tablespoons of Milk of Magnesia. Since a medicine cup was available, he poured the Milk of Magnesia up to the _____ dram calibration line.

10. A 20 Kg child was to receive Cosmegen, 15 mcg/Kg of body weight. The child should receive _____ mcg or _____ mg.

11. A pregnant woman was prescribed 60 mg of Fergon daily. Her cumulative monthly dose (30 days) would be approximately _____ grams.

12. A patient who receives 3 teaspoons or 1 tablespoon of Kayexalate, four times per day, would be receiving a daily dose equivalent to _____ ounces.

13. A patient takes Aldomet, 500 mg tablets, 3 to 4 times per day. He is advised not to exceed a daily dose of 3 grams or _____ tablets.

Unit III

Dosage Calculation

Accurate dosage calculations are an essential component of the total nursing role in the safe administration of medications. This section will present common dosage calculations necessary for preparing medications for the oral and parenteral routes.

Chapter 9

Oral Dosages

The oral route is a simple, economic method of drug delivery that is safe and convenient for the systemic administration of medications by mouth.

When the prescribed or desired drug dosage is different from what is available or "on-hand," a dosage calculation is necessary to determine the amount of drug to give. The easiest formula to work with is:

$$\frac{\text{desired amount}}{\text{on-hand}} \times \text{quantity} = \text{amount to give}$$

This formula works well when calculating dosages *in the same system*. The symbol Rx is used throughout to indicate the desired amount.

Dosage Problems for Medications in the Same System

EXAMPLE: Rx: 0.250 mg digoxin

On-hand: 0.125 mg
                digoxin/tablet

Give: _____ tablet(s)

Use Formula: $\dfrac{\text{desired amount}}{\text{on-hand}} \times \text{quantity}$

$= \text{amount to give}$

$\dfrac{0.250 \text{ mg}}{0.125 \text{ mg}} = 0.250 \div 0.125 = 2$

$2 \times \text{quantity (1 tablet)} = 2$
Give 2 tablets.

EXAMPLE: Rx: 100 mg of phenobarbital
elixir
On-hand: 20 mg/5 ml
Give: _____ ml

Use Formula: $\dfrac{\text{desired amount}}{\text{on-hand}} \times \text{quantity}$
$= \text{amount to give}$

$\dfrac{100 \text{ mg}}{20 \text{ mg}} = 100 \div 20 = 5$

$5 \times \text{quantity (5 ml)} = 25$

Give 25 ml.

Practice Problems

1. Furosemide (Lasix) 160 mg daily is prescribed. Lasix 40 mg tablets are on-hand. Give
_____ tablet(s).

2. Trilisate 1500 mg is prescribed. Trilisate liquid is labeled 500 mg per 15 ml. Give
_____ ml.

3. Allopurinal 150 mg is prescribed. Allopurinal 300 mg tablets are on-hand. Give _____ tablet(s).

4. Codeine elixir 20 mg is prescribed. Codeine elixir is labeled 10 mg per 5 ml. Give _____ ml.

5. Brethine 7.5 mg is prescribed, T.I.D. Brethine 2.5 mg tablets are on-hand. Give _____ tablet(s), T.I.D.

6. Demerol 100 mg is prescribed, every 4 to 6 hours, as needed. Demerol 50 mg tablets are on-hand. Give _____ tablet(s) for each dose.

7. Phenobarbital Elixir 75 mg is prescribed. Phenobarbital Elixir is labeled 20 mg per 5 ml. Give _____ ml.

8. Hydrodiuril 25 mg is prescribed. Hydrodiuril 50 mg tablets are on-hand. Give _____ tablet(s).

9. Synthroid 0.30 mg is prescribed. Synthroid 0.015 mg tablets are on-hand. Give _____ tablet(s).

10. Coumadin 15 mg is prescribed. Coumadin 10 mg tablets are on-hand. Give _____ tablet(s).

11. Mellaril 75 mg is prescribed. T.I.D. Mellaril 25 mg tablets are on-hand. Give _____ tablet(s).

12. Dilantin 300 mg is prescribed. Dilantin suspension is labeled 125 mg per 5 ml. Give _____ ml.

Dosage Problems for Medication in Different Systems

■ **RULE: Whenever the desired and on-hand drug dosages are in different systems you would:**

1. Choose the approximate equivalent.
2. Use ratio and proportion to solve for x.
3. Use the formula D/H × Q = amount to give, if necessary.

EXAMPLE: Rx: 0.8 grams of Anturance daily
Give: _____ grains daily

Equivalent: 1 gram = 15 grains

Complete the Proportion: 1 gram:15 grains::0.8 grams:x grains

1 gram × x grains = 0.8 grams × 15 grains

$1x = 0.8 × 15$

$1x = 12$

Solve for x:

$$\frac{1x}{1} = \frac{12}{1}$$

$$\frac{\cancel{1}x}{\cancel{1}} = \frac{12}{1}$$

$$x = 12$$

Answer = 12 grains

EXAMPLE: Rx: 500 mg Gantrisin, Q.I.D.

On-hand: 0.5 gram tablets
Give: _____ tablet(s)

Change: To change 500 milligrams to grams move the decimal point (500. mg) three places to the left, .500.. Then 500 mg = 0.5 grams.

Use: $\dfrac{\text{desired amount}}{\text{on-hand}} \times \text{quantity}$

= amount to give

$\dfrac{0.5 \text{ grams}}{0.5 \text{ grams}} = 1$

$1 \times \text{quantity (1 tablet)} = 1$

Answer = 1 tablet

EXAMPLE: Rx: 45 cc Elixophyllin elixir
Give: _____ fluidrams

Equivalent: 30 cc = 8 f℥

Complete the Proportion: 30 cc:8 f℥ :: 45 cc:x f℥
30 cc × x f℥ = 45 cc × 8 f℥

Solve for x: $30x = 45 \times 8$

$30x = 360$

$\dfrac{30x}{30} = \dfrac{360}{30}$

$\dfrac{\overset{1}{\cancel{30}}\, x}{\underset{1}{\cancel{30}}} = \dfrac{\overset{12}{\cancel{360}}}{\underset{1}{\cancel{30}}}$

$x = 12 \text{ f℥}$

Answer = 12 f℥

EXAMPLE: Rx: morphine sulfate grain $\frac{1}{4}$

On-hand: morphine sulfate 10 mg tablets

Give: _____ tablet(s)

Equivalent: 1 grain = 60 mg

Complete the Proportion: 1 grain:60 mg :: $\frac{1}{4}$ grain:x mg

1 grain $\times x$ mg = $\frac{1}{4}$ grain $\times$ 60 mg

Solve for x: $1x = \frac{1}{4} \times 60$

$1x = 15$

$\frac{1x}{1} = \frac{15}{1}$

$\frac{\cancel{1}x}{\cancel{1}} = \frac{15}{1}$

$x = 15$ mg

Use: $\dfrac{\text{desired amount}}{\text{on-hand}} \times \text{quantity}$

= amount to give

$\dfrac{15 \text{ mg}}{10 \text{ mg}} = 15 \div 10 = 1.5$

1.5 × quantity (1 tablet)

$$= 1.5 \text{ or } 1\frac{1}{2} \text{tablets}$$

$$Answer = 1\frac{1}{2}\text{tablets}$$

Practice Problems

1. Depakene 0.75 grams is prescribed. Depakene syrup is labeled 250 mg per 5 ml. Give _____ ml.

2. Zarontin syrup 0.5 grams is prescribed. Zarontin syrup is labeled 250 mg per 5 ml. Give _____ ml.

3. Peganone 2 grams is prescribed in four equally divided portions. Peganone 500 mg tablets are on-hand. Give _____ tablet(s) each time.

4. Thorazine hydrochloride is on-hand in a syrup (3 mg/ml). The prescribed dose is 3 teaspoons. Give _____ ml, which would be equal to _____ mg.

5. NegGram is on-hand in 0.5-gram tablets. The prescribed dose is grains 30, Q.I.D. Give _____ tablet(s), Q.I.D.

6. Scopolamine hydrobromide is on-hand in 0.6-mg tablets. The prescribed dose is grains 1/100. Give _____ tablet(s).

7. Tylenol gr X is prescribed. Tylenol elixir is labeled 160 mg per teaspoon. Give _____ ml.

8. Choledyl 0.25 gm is prescribed. Choledyl Elixir is labeled 100 mg per 5 ml. Give _____ ml.

9. Colchicine 1.2 mg is prescribed. Colchicine gr 1/100 is on-hand. Give _____ tablet(s).

10. Pen-Vee K 2 grams is prescribed. Pen-Vee K 500 mg tablets are on-hand. Give _____ tablet(s).

11. Proloid is on-hand in gr 1/4 tablets. The prescribed dose is 60 mg. Give _____ tablets.

12. Amoxicillin 0.5 gm is prescribed every eight hours. Amoxicillin oral suspension is labeled 250 mg/teaspoon. Give _____ ml.

13. Tigan 250 mg is prescribed. Tigan 100 mg tablets are on-hand. Give _____ tablet(s).

14. Provera 10 mg is prescribed. Provera 2.5 mg tablets are on-hand. Give _____ tablet(s).

15. Motrin 0.8 gm is prescribed. Motrin 400 mg tablets are on-hand. Give _____ tablet(s).

End of Chapter Review

Solve the following problems:

1. Coumadin sodium 30 mg daily is prescribed. Coumadin sodium 10-mg tablets are on-hand. Give _____ tablet(s).

2. Ascorbic acid 300 mg is prescribed. Ascorbic acid 100-mg tablets are on-hand. Give _____ tablet(s).

3. Mysaline 1.5 grams daily is prescribed. Mysaline liquid is labeled 250 mg per 5 ml. Give _____ ml.

4. Hydrodiuril 0.2 grams is prescribed. Hydrodiuril 50 mg tablets are on-hand. Give _____ tablet(s).

5. Atropine sulfate is on-hand in 0.3 mg tablets. The prescribed dose is grain 1/200. Give _____ tablet(s).

6. Serax is available in 15-mg tablets. The prescribed daily dose is grains 1/2. Give _____ tablet(s).

7. Cephulac 20 grams is prescribed. Cephulac 30 grams in 45 ml is on-hand. Give _____ ounces.

8. Nitroglycerin grains 1/150 is prescribed. Nitroglycerin 0.4 mg tablets are on-hand. Give _____ tablet(s).

9. Morphine Sulfate grains 1/4 is prescribed. Morphine Sulfate Oral Solution is labeled 10 mg per 5 ml. Give _____ ml.

Chapter 10

Parenteral Dosages

The term *parenteral* refers to any route of drug delivery other than the digestive tract (enteral route). Parenteral commonly refers to the injection of drugs into body tissues (using a needle and syringe) and into body fluids. *Needle precautions should always be followed*. Parenteral drugs must be sterile and should absorb easily without causing tissue irritation.

The parenteral route is recommended if a medication would be ineffectively absorbed in the gastrointestinal tract or take too long to become effective. Parenteral drugs are administered in the form of sterile liquid preparations.

Dosage calculations can be solved by using ratio and proportion or by using the formula:

$$\frac{\text{desired amount}}{\text{on-hand}} \times \text{quantity} = \text{amount to give}$$

For those of you who wish to review information about the various parenteral routes, please refer to Appendices B through F. Although this material is not specifically math-related, it has been included for your convenience.

Dosage Problems for Medications in the Same System

EXAMPLE: Rx: 1.0 mg folic acid

On-hand: 5.0 mg/ml folic acid

Give: _____ ml

Use Formula: $\dfrac{\text{desired amount}}{\text{on-hand}} \times \text{quantity} \left\{ \dfrac{D}{H} \times Q \right.$

= amount to give

$$\frac{1.0 \text{ mg}}{5.0 \text{ mg}} = \frac{1}{5}$$

$$\frac{1}{5} \times \text{quantity (1 ml)} = 0.20 \text{ ml}$$

Answer = 0.2 ml

EXAMPLE: Rx: 150 mg lincomycin

On-hand: 300 mg/ml lincomycin

Give: _____ ml

Use Formula: $\dfrac{\text{desired amount}}{\text{on-hand}} \times \text{quantity} \left\{ \dfrac{D}{H} \times Q \right.$

= amount to give

$$\frac{150 \text{ mg}}{300 \text{ mg}} = \frac{1}{2}$$

$$\frac{1}{2} \times \text{quantity (1 ml)} = 0.50 \text{ ml}$$

Answer = 0.5 ml

Dosage Problems for Medications in Different Systems

Whenever the desired and on-hand drug dosages are in different systems you would:

1. Choose the equivalent.
2. Use ratio and proportion to solve for x.
3. Use the formula D/H × Q = amount to give, if necessary.

EXAMPLE: The physician requested gr iss of Garamycin to be administered IM, b.i.d. The on-hand medication was labeled 60 mg per ml. The nurse would administer _____ ml, b.i.d.

Equivalent: 1 grain = 60 milligrams

Complete the Proportion: 1 grain:60 mg :: $1\frac{1}{2}$ grains:x mg

$$1 \text{ grain} \times x \text{ mg} = 1\frac{1}{2} \text{ grains} \times 60 \text{ mg}$$

Solve for x:
$$1x = 1\frac{1}{2} \times 60$$

$$1x = \frac{3}{2_1} \times \overset{30}{60} = 90$$

$$x = 90 \text{ mg}$$

Use: $\dfrac{\text{D}}{\text{H}} \times \text{Q}$ $\Big\}$ $\qquad \dfrac{\text{desired amount}}{\text{on-hand}} \times \text{quantity}$
$$= \text{amount to give}$$

$$\frac{90 \text{ mg}}{60 \text{ mg}} = \frac{3}{2}$$

$$\frac{3}{2} \times 1 \text{ ml} = 1\frac{1}{2} \text{ ml}$$

$$\textit{Answer} = 1\frac{1}{2} \text{ ml}$$

Medications Packaged as Powders

The available amount of drug is in a solute form (dry powder) and needs to be reconstituted by adding a dilutent (solvent). The label on the available drug will give directions for adding the dilutent. There are three common dilutents that must always be sterile when added to the dry powder. Use one of the three:

- Bacteriostatic water
- Sodium chloride (0.9%)
- Sterile water

Read labeled directions for reconstitution:

- Recommended dilutent
- Quantity of dilutent
- Ratio of solute to solvent after reconstitution

Use $\dfrac{\text{desired amount}}{\text{on-hand}} \times \text{quantity} = \text{amount to give}$

EXAMPLE: The physician prescribed 250 mg of Ancef, IM, every 8 hours. The medication was available as a powder in a 1-gram vial.

Reconstitute: Labeled directions: Reconstitute with 2.5 ml of Sterile Water for Injection. Shake well until dissolved. Solution concentration will equal 330 mg per ml. Fluid volume will equal 3.0 ml.

Dissolve 1 gram powder with 2.5 ml of sterile water.

Use:

$$\frac{\text{desired amount}}{\text{on-hand}} \times \text{quantity} = \text{amount to give}$$

$$\frac{250 \text{ mg}}{1000 \text{ mg*}} = \frac{1}{4}$$

$$\frac{1}{4} \times 3.0 \text{ ml} = 0.75 \text{ ml or } \frac{3}{4} \text{ ml}$$

$$Answer = \frac{3}{4} \text{ ml}$$

Practice Problems

1. The physician requested that a patient receive 0.002 grams of folic acid, IM, per day, for five days, for severe intestinal malabsorption. The injection was on-hand as 1.0 mg/ml. The nurse would give _____ ml a day for five days.

*Approximate quantity (330 mg/1.0 ml = 990 mg/3.0).

2. The physician requested that 120 mg of furo-semide be administered IM in three equally divided doses every 8 hours for 2 days. The drug was available for injections as 10 mg/ml. The nurse should give _____ ml every 8 hours.

3. Robaxin 0.3 grams IM was prescribed. The drug was on-hand as 100 mg/ml for injection. The nurse would give _____ ml.

4. Compazine 15 mg IM is prescribed for severe nausea and vomiting. Compazine is available as 5 mg/ml. The nurse should give _____ ml.

5. Haldrol 4 mg IM was prescribed. Haldrol was on-hand as 5 mg/ml. The nurse should give _____ ml.

End of Chapter Review

1. Aldomet 125 mg was prescribed, IM, q.i.d. The medication was available for injecting as 250 mg/5 ml. The nurse would administer _____ ml, q.i.d.

2. Valium 2 mg was prescribed, IM, p.r.n., every 3 to 4 hours. The medication was available for injection as 5 mg/ml. The nurse would give _____ ml every 3 to 4 hours as needed.

3. The physician requested that a patient receive 1.5 mg of Stadol, IM, every 3 to 4 hours

as needed for pain. The medication was available for injection as 2.0 mg/ml. The nurse would give _____ ml every 3 to 4 hours, p.r.n.

4. Demerol 35 mg, IM, is prescribed for pain. Demerol was available for injection as 50 mg/ml. The nurse would give _____ ml.

5. The physican prescribed 6 mg of AquaME-PHYTON, IM, weekly. The medication was available as 2 mg/ml. The nurse would give _____ ml every week.

6. Versed 3 mg, IM is prescribed preoperatively to induce drowsiness. Versed was available as 5 mg/ml. The nurse would give _____ ml.

7. The physician prescribed Dilaudid 3 mg, IM, every 4 to 6 hours for analgesia. Dilaudid is available as 4 mg/ml. The nurse would give _____ ml every 4 to 6 hours.

8. Lasix 30 mg, IM is prescribed as a diuretic. Lasix was available as 40 mg/ml. The nurse would give _____ ml.

9. Atropine 0.5 mg was ordered preoperatively, subcutaneously. The medication was available in a vial as grains 1/150 per 1.0 ml. The nurse would give _____ ml.

10. Scopolamine 0.3 mg was ordered subcutaneously as a preanesthetic medication. The medication was available in ampules containing

grains 1/200 per ml. The nurse would give
_____ ml.

11. The physician prescribed Morphine Sulfate
grains 1/5 IM every 4 to 6 hours for severe
pain. The medication was available as 15 mg/
ml. The nurse would give _____ ml, every 4 to
6 hours, as needed.

12. The physician prescribed grains iii of Seconal,
IM. The medication was available as 100 mg/
ml for injection. The nurse would give _____
ml.

13. The physician prescribed 500 mg of Cefizox,
IM, every 12 hours for a genitourinary infection. The medication was available as a powder in a 2-gram vial. Reconstitute with 6.0 ml
of Sterile Water for Injection and shake well.
Solution concentration will provide 270 mg/
ml. Fluid volume will equal 7.4 ml. Use approximate quantities for dosage calculations.
Give _____ ml every 12 hours.

14. Methicillin sodium 1.5 grams, IM, was prescribed for a systemic infection. Four (4)
grams of the medication was available as a
powder in a vial. Directions state to reconstitute with 5.7 ml of Sterile Water for Injection
and shake well. Solution concentration will
provide 500 mg/ml. To give 1.5 grams the
nurse would give _____ ml.

15. The physician prescribed 400 mg of Solu-Cortef, IM, for severe inflammation. The medication was available as a powder in a 2-gram vial. Reconstitute according to directions so that each 8 ml will contain 7 grams of Solu-Cortef. The nurse would then give _____ ml to give 400 mg.

16. The physician prescribed 1.0 mg, IM, of leucovorin calcium, once a day, for the treatment of megaloblastic anemia. The medication was available as a powder in a 50-mg vial. Reconstitute with 5.0 ml of Bacteriostatic Water for Injection. Shake well. Solution concentration will yield 10 mg/ml. Fluid volume will equal 5.0 ml. Give _____ ml, once a day.

Chapter 11

Drugs Measured in Units

Drugs are measured in units when strength can be more accurately determined than weight. There are three major drugs that are measured in units: heparin, penicillin, and insulin. Dosage calculations for heparin and penicillin are solved using this formula: D/H × Q = amount to give.

Heparin

■ **RULE: To Prepare Heparin for Injection, Follow These Steps:**

- Read the medication order, noting the number of units to be administered. For example, a patient is prescribed 5000 units of heparin to be administered subcutaneously every 12 hours.
- Select the appropriate ampule/vial. For example, you choose a 10 ml multi-dose vial in a concentration of 20,000 units/ml.
- Choose a 1.0 ml syringe.

Use Formula: $\dfrac{\text{desired amount}}{\text{on-hand}} \times \text{quantity} = \text{amount to give}$

$$\frac{5000 \text{ U}}{20{,}000 \text{ U}} = \frac{1}{4}$$

$$\frac{1}{4} \times 1.0 \text{ ml (quantity)} = 0.25 \text{ ml}$$

Answer = 0.25 ml

Heparin sodium lock flush solution contains a small dose of heparin and is used to maintain the patency of intravenous catheters. The hep-lock flush solution contains 10 or 100 units/milliliter. It is administered after a normal saline flush, which follows administration of an intravenous medication, usually an antibiotic. Winthrop has manufactured a Hep-Pak® convenience package for heparin lock flush procedures. The Hep-Pak® contains one cartridge of heparin lock flush solution (10–100 U/ml) and two cartridges of sodium chloride solution.

Penicillin

Some preparations of penicillin come in units/ml, whereas others come in milligrams/ml. You can use ratio and proportion or the formula D/H × Q = amount to give.

■ **RULE: To Prepare Penicillin for Injection, Follow These Steps:**

■ Read the medication order, noting the number of units to be administered. For example, a patient is prescribed 300,000 units of penicillin G procaine to be administered q 12 hours.

■ Penicillin G procaine is available as 600,000 units/1.2 ml. Therefore you would use the formula D/H × Q = Amount:

$$\frac{\text{desired}}{\text{on-hand}} \times \text{quantity} = \text{amount to give}$$

EXAMPLE: $\frac{300,000 \text{ U}}{600,000 \text{ U}} = \frac{3}{6} = \frac{1}{2}$

$\frac{1}{2} \times 1.2 \text{ ml} = 0.6 \text{ ml}$

Answer = 0.6 ml

Insulin

It is easy to prepare insulin for injection. Insulin is packaged in vials of 100 units/ml (U = 100/ml) and the insulin syringe is calibrated in 100 units/ml. Medication orders are written in units/ml. Therefore, all you have to do is draw up the desired dose by filling the insulin syringe to the identified calibration. Mathematical calculations are not required.

■ RULE: **To Prepare Insulin for Injection, Follow These Steps:**

■ Read the medication order, noting the type of insulin and unit preparation desired. For example, a patient is ordered 30 units of regular insulin.
■ Select the insulin. Check the label three times. You would choose the vial of Iletin (regular) insulin marked 100 units/ml.

- Match the insulin syringe to the unit preparation of insulin. You should choose a U-100
  syringe since the insulin preparation comes
  in a vial marked 100 U/ml.
- Draw up the required dose by filling the syringe to the desired calibration. You would
  fill a U-100 syringe to the 30 units calibration
  (see Figure 11–1).

Insulin Delivery Systems

Insulin is also available for injection in 1.5-ml cartridges (100 units/ml [U 100]) for use with
NovoPen® and Novolin Pen® insulin delivery systems. (See Figure 11–2.) The insulin delivery devices look like a fountain pen, are about 6 inches
long, weigh 5 to 7 ounces, and are designed for
patients to give themselves insulin by using a
pushbutton/plunger mechanism. Both systems
use PenNeedle® disposable needles and Novolin®
insulin; Regular, NPH, or a combination of NPH
(70%) and Regular (30%). Medication orders are
written in insulin units. Mathematical calculations
are not required. Your responsibilities include:
assessing the patient's ability to assemble the
equipment and helping the patient with it as necessary, checking the accuracy of the dose delivered, evaluating the patient's response to the
medication, and documenting that the dosage

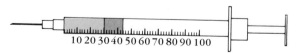

Figure 11–1. Shaded area indicates 30 units of
regular insulin in a U-100 syringe.

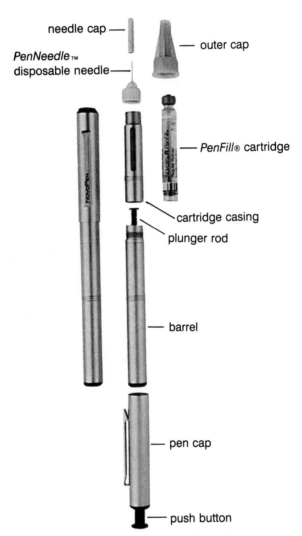

needle cap

PenNeedle™
disposable needle

outer cap

PenFill® cartridge

cartridge casing

plunger rod

barrel

pen cap

push button

Figure 11–2. NovoPen® Insulin Delivery System.
Courtesy of Novo Nordisk Pharmaceuticals Inc.

was given as prescribed. You should refer to product literature (available from Squibb-Novo, Inc.*) for specific instructions on assembly and injection.

Mixing Two Types of Insulin

Frequently you will find it necessary to mix two types of insulin, usually regular and NPH. When you have to mix insulins there are two important guidelines that you must remember:

1. Do not contaminate the contents of one vial with the contents of the other vial.
2. Always *draw up the NPH insulin last* because chemically it has a protein substance in it that regular insulin does not have. Drawing up the NPH insulin last helps prevent contamination of the regular insulin.

■ RULE: **To Prepare Two Types of Insulin for Injection, Regular and NPH, Follow These Steps:**

- Wash your hands and obtain the correct vials of insulin and the correct syringes. Both should be in the same unit of strength (U-100).
- Wipe the top of both vials with an alcohol swab.

*Squibb-Novo, Inc., 211 Carnegie Center, Princeton, NJ 08549-6213. (609) 987-5800.

- Inject air equal to the insulin dose of NPH (20 units) into the NPH insulin vial first (*A*). *Do not touch the insulin with the needle.* Withdraw the needle.
- Inject air equal to the dose of regular insulin (30 units) into the regular insulin (*B*). Be careful that the needle does not touch the solution because air should not be bubbled through the solution.

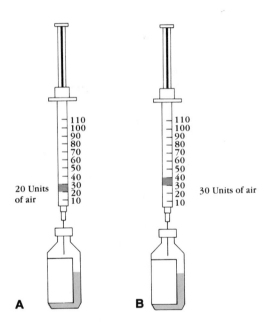

20 Units of air

30 Units of air

A
B

- Invert the vial of regular insulin and draw back the required dosage (*C*). Check the dosage (30 units).
- Remove the needle from the vial of regular insulin (*D*).

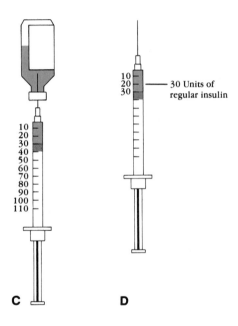

30 Units of regular insulin

C   **D**

- Put the needle into the NPH vial (*E*).
- Invert and draw back the required dosage (20 units). There will now be a total of 50 units (*F*).

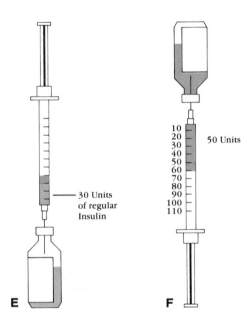

E — 30 Units of regular Insulin

F — 50 Units

■ Check the dose (*G*) and check for air bubbles. Cap the needle and prepare to administer.

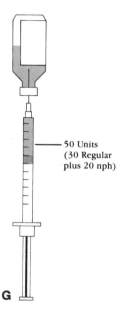

50 Units
(30 Regular
plus 20 nph)

G

End of Chapter Review

1. A patient is to receive 10,000 units of heparin subcutaneously at 8:00 a.m. and 8:00 p.m. for 5 days. Heparin sodium for injection is available in a TUBEX Cartridge-Needle unit in 15,000 units per ml. The nurse would give _____ ml every 12 hours.

2. The physician prescribed 5000 units of heparin for injection intravenously through a heparin lock. Heparin is available in a 10-ml vial in a concentration of 20,000 units per milliliter. The nurse would administer _____ ml.

3. Heparin sodium, 8000 units, is prescribed subcutaneously, every 8 hours. The medication is available in a vial labeled 10,000 units per milliliter. The nurse would give _____ ml, every 8 hours.

4. The physician prescribed heparin sodium, 5000 units, subcutaneously, twice a day. Heparin is available in a vial labeled 7,500 units per milliliter. The nurse would give _____ ml, twice a day.

5. The physician prescribed 300,000 units of Bicillin intramuscularly every 12 hours for 5 days. Bicillin is packaged as 600,000 units/ml. The nurse would give _____ ml every 12 hours.

6. The physician prescribed penicillin G potassium 125,000 units, IM, every 12 hours. The medication is available in solution as 250,000 units/5 ml. The nurse would give _____ ml every 12 hours.

7. Penicillin G benzathine 1.2 million units was prescribed, IM, as a single injection. The medication is available as 300,000 units per milliliter. The nurse would give _____ ml.

8. The physician prescribed Crysticillin 600,000 units IM as a single dose. Crysticillin is available in a 12-ml vial labeled 500,000 units per milliliter. The nurse would give _____ ml.

9. The physician prescribed 15 units of U-100 regular insulin subcutaneously at 11:00 a.m. to cover a sugar and acetone reading of + 1. The nurse had a U-100 syringe. She would draw up into the syringe _____ units.

10. The physician prescribed 50 units of Hummulin N insulin subcutaneously at 8:00 a.m. Using a U-100 insulin syringe, the nurse would draw up _____ units.

11. The physician prescribed a combination of 22 units of NPH insulin and 12 units of regular insulin. Using a U-100 insulin syringe, the nurse would draw up a total of _____ units, making certain to draw up the _____ insulin last.

12. To help a patient give himself 6 units of Novolin® insulin using a NovoPen®, the nurse would remind the patient to depress the push button _____ times since each depression releases _____ units of insulin.

Chapter 12

Immunostimulants: Vaccines, Toxoids, and Immune Serum Globulins

Vaccines and Toxoids contain particles of bacteria or viruses that have been killed or are less virulent than the original pathogen. They provide *active immunity* by triggering an immune response that would occur if a person had become infected. Examples include: DPT triple antigen, Hepatitis B vaccine, rabies vaccine, and Poliovirus vaccine. Research is ongoing in an effort to develop an AIDS vaccine. Immune serum globulins provide *passive immunity* by supplying antibodies from a previously infected source to a person who may or has been exposed to an infectious agent. Examples include: Immune serum globulin, Hepatitis B immune globulin, and RhoGAM.

Immunostimulants are available in milliliters or international units (IU) and are administered intradermally, subcutaneously, and intramuscularly. Rules for drug preparation can be found in Chapters 10 and 11. Appendices B, C, and D will provide a helpful review of technique.

End of Chapter Review

1. A physician prescribed 0.5 ml of Hibivax, subcutaneously, for a 4-year-old. The nurse

should reconstitute with 6 ml of the diluent provided by the manufacturer. The vial will provide 10 doses. The nurse would give _____ ml.

2. A patient is to receive 0.5 ml of rubella virus vaccine, subcutaneously. Reconstitute, using the entire amount of dilutent supplied by the manufacturer. The nurse would give _____ ml.

3. A physician prescribes rabies immune globulin, 20 units/kg, IM, for a patient who weighs 145 pounds. The rabies immune globulin is labeled 150 units/ml. The nurse would give _____ ml.

4. A patient is to receive 500 units of tetanus immune globulin, IM. The medication is available as 250 units/ml. The nurse would give _____ ml.

5. The nurse is to administer 625 units of varicellazoster immune globulin, IM. The medication is labeled 125 units/2.5 ml. The nurse would give _____ ml.

6. Hepatitis B immune globulin 0.06 ml/kg is prescribed IM for a patient who weighs 110 pounds. The nurse would give _____ ml.

7. The physician prescribed immune globulin 0.25 ml/kg, IM for post-exposure prophylaxis of measles. The patient weighs 119 pounds. The nurse would give _____ ml.

8. The physician prescribed 25 mg, IM, of Hib-Imune. Hib-Imune is labeled 25 mg/0.5 ml. The drug requires reconstitution with the dilutent provided by the manufacturer. To give 25 mg, the nurse would give _____ ml.

Chapter 13

Pediatric and Geriatric Dosages and Nursing Considerations

Pediatric Dosages

Infants and children cannot receive the same dose of medication as adults. This is because a child's physiologic immaturity influences how a drug is absorbed, excreted, distributed, and used. Pediatric dosages are based on age, body weight, or body surface area. If you are going to be giving pediatric drugs, you must become familiar with the following rules for calculating pediatric dosages.

Rules Based on Age

■ FRIED'S RULE: **For Newborns to 2-Year-Olds**

- Determine the child's age in months.
- Divide the age in months by 150.
- Multiply by the adult dose.
- Use $\dfrac{\text{Age (in months)}}{150} \times$ normal adult dose.
- If necessary, use $\dfrac{\text{desired amount}}{\text{on-hand}} \times$ quantity = amount to give.

EXAMPLE: The physician prescribed Dolanex elixir for a 15-month-old. The normal adult dose is 325 mg every 4 to 6 hours. Dolanex elixir is available as 325 mg/5 ml.

Use:

Fried's Rule: Pediatric dose

$$= \frac{\text{age in months}}{150}$$

$\times$ normal adult dose

$$\text{Pediatric dose} = \frac{15 \text{ months}}{150}$$

$$= \frac{1}{10} \times 325 \text{ mg} = 32.5 \text{ mg}$$

Because Dolanex is available as 325 mg/5 ml, additional computation is necessary to determine the amount of milliliters to give.

Use:

$$\frac{\text{desired amount}}{\text{on-hand}} \times \text{quantity}$$

$$= \text{amount to give}$$

$$\frac{32.5 \text{ mg}}{325 \text{ mg}} = \frac{1}{10}$$

$$\frac{1}{10} \times 5.0 \text{ ml} = 0.5 \text{ ml}$$

Answer $= 0.5$ ml

- ■ **Young's Rule:**
For Children Ages 1 to 12

  - ■ Determine the child's age in years.
  - ■ Divide the age in years by the age in years + 12.
  - ■ Multiply by the adult dose.
  - ■ Use $\dfrac{\text{age (in years)}}{\text{age (in years)} + 12} \times$ normal adult dose.
  - ■ If necessary, use $\dfrac{\text{desired amount}}{\text{on-hand}} \times$ quantity = amount to give.

EXAMPLE: The physician prescribed Milk of Magnesia for an 8-year-old patient. The normal adult dose is 30 ml.

Use: *Young's Rule:* Pediatric dose

$$= \frac{\text{age (in years)}}{\text{age} + 12}$$

$\times$ normal adult dose

$$\text{Pediatric dose} = \frac{8}{8 + 12}$$

$$= \frac{8}{20} = \frac{2}{\underset{1}{5}} \times \overset{6}{30} \text{ ml} = 12 \text{ ml}$$

Answer = 12 ml

EXAMPLE: A physician prescribed Dolanex elixir for a 4-year-old. The normal adult dose is 325 mg every 4 to 6 hours. Dolanex elixir is available as 325 mg/5 ml.

Young's Rule: Pediatric dose

Use:
$$= \frac{\text{age (in years)}}{\text{age (in years)} + 12}$$
$$\times \text{ normal adult dose.}$$

$$\text{Pediatric dose} = \frac{4}{4 + 12} = \frac{4}{16}$$

$$= \frac{1}{4} \times 325 \text{ mg} = 81 \text{ mg}$$

Use:
$$\frac{\text{desired amount}}{\text{on-hand}} \times \text{quantity}$$
$$= \text{amount to give}$$

$$\frac{81 \text{ mg}}{325 \text{ mg}} = \frac{1}{4} \text{(approximate)}$$
$$\frac{1}{4} \times 5.0 \text{ ml} = 1.25 \text{ ml}$$

Answer = 1.25 ml

Rules Based on Weight

■ **CLARK'S RULE: For 2-Year-Olds and Older Children**

- Determine the child's weight in pounds.
- Divide the weight by 150.
- Multiply by the normal adult dose.
- Use $\frac{\text{weight in pounds}}{150} \times$ normal adult dose.
- If necessary, use $\frac{\text{desired amount}}{\text{on-hand}} \times$ quantity
  = amount to give.

EXAMPLE: The physician prescribed Dolanex elixir for a 4-year-old who weighs 30 pounds. The normal adult dose is 325 mg every 4 to 6 hours. Dolanex elixir is available as 325 mg/5 ml.

Use: *Clark's Rule:* Pediatric dose

$$= \frac{\text{weight in pounds}}{150}$$

$\times$ normal adult dose.

$$\text{Pediatric dose} = \frac{30}{150} = \frac{1}{5}$$

$$\frac{1}{5} \times 325 \text{ mg} = 65 \text{ mg}$$

Use: $\dfrac{\text{desired amount}}{\text{on-hand}} \times \text{quantity}$

$= \text{amount to give}$

$$\frac{65 \text{ mg}}{325 \text{ mg}} = \frac{1}{5}$$

$$\frac{1}{5} \times 5 \text{ ml} = 1.0 \text{ ml}$$

Answer = 1.0 ml

Sometimes medications are prescribed in milligrams/kilogram of body weight. Since there are 2.2 pounds in a kilogram, you must convert the child's weight in pounds to kilograms before you can calculate the drug dosage. The rule below tells you how to calculate drug dosages when the drug is ordered according to kilograms of body weight.

■ RULE: **To Change Pounds to Kilograms, Follow These Steps:**

- Determine the patient's body weight in pounds.
- Divide by 2.2.
- Solve the problem using the appropriate rule.

EXAMPLE: The physician prescribed 20 mg of amoxicillin/kg of body weight to be administered q 8 hours in equally divided doses. The patient weighed 44 pounds and was 5 years old. Divide by 2.2 to determine body weight in kilograms.

$$2.2. \overline{)44.0.}$$

Move the decimal point in the divisor and the dividend the same number of places. Put the decimal point directly above the line for the quotient.

$$\frac{20.}{22)440} \text{(quotient)}$$

Answer = 20 kg

Use: Use a proportion to solve for *x*.

$$20 \text{ mg}:1 \text{ kg}::x \text{ mg}:20 \text{ kg}$$

$$1x = 20 \times 20$$

$$1x = 400$$

$$x = 400 \text{ mg}$$

400 mg will be divided into three equal doses. 400 mg ÷ 3 = 133 mg to be given every 8 hours.

Answer = 133 mg

Rule Based on Body Surface Area

Basing a pediatric dosage on body surface area is the most accurate way of determining the amount of drug to give.

■ **RULE: To Determine a Pediatric Dosage Based on Body Surface Area, Follow These Steps:**

- Estimate the child's body surface area in square meters (m²). Refer to a nomogram (Figure 13–1)*
- Use:

$$\frac{\text{child's surface area in square meters}}{1.73 \text{ m}^2 \text{ (surface area of an average adult)}}$$

$\times$ adult dose

*The nomogram is used to determine body surface area. To use the nomograms in Figure 13–1, you need to draw a straight line from the patient's height to his weight. You will intersect the body surface column at a number that indicates the patient's body surface area in square meters (m²). See page 161.

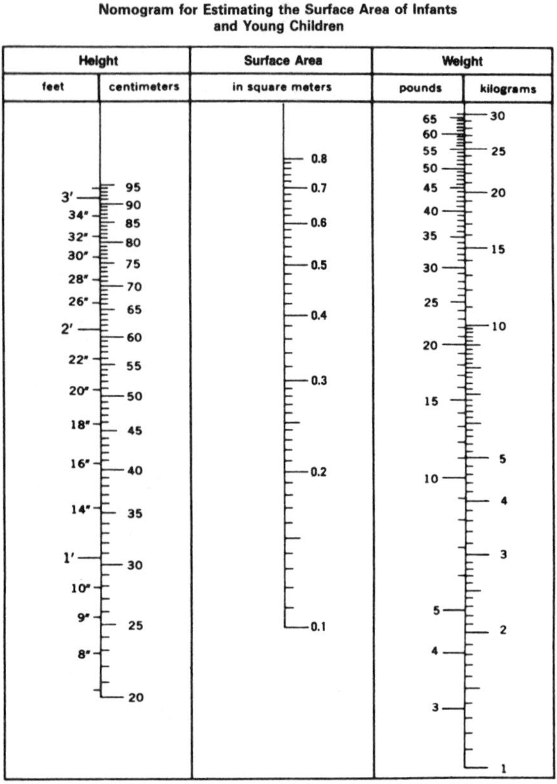

Figure 13-1. Nomograms for estimating surface area of body. Nomogram on opposite page indicates 1.05 m² surface area for a child who weighs 75 pounds and is 4 feet, 2 inches tall. (Illustrations courtesy Abbott Laboratories, North Chicago, IL)

**Nomogram for Estimating the Surface Area
of Older Children and Adults**

Height		Surface Area	Weight	
feet	centimeters	in square meters	pounds	kilograms

■ If necessary, use a proportion to solve for x.

EXAMPLE: The physician prescribed Benadryl 150 mg/m²/day, for an 8-year-old child who weighs 75 pounds and is 50 inches tall (4 feet, 2 inches). The normal adult dose is 25 mg, q.i.d. The nurse would give _____ mg q.i.d.

Use: Body Surface Area Rule:

$$\frac{\text{child's surface area in square meters (m}^2)}{1.73 \text{ m}^2}$$

$\times$ adult dose

$$\frac{1.05 \text{ m}^2}{1.73 \text{ m}^2} = 0.60 \times 25 \text{ mg} = 15.17 \text{ mg}$$

To prepare Benadryl for administration it would be best to drop the .17 and prepare 15 mg.

Answer = 15 mg, q.i.d.

Nursing Concerns for Pediatric Drug Administration

When administering medications to children, you need to be aware of the following:

■ Explain honestly what will be done; explain at the level of the child's understanding.
■ Use supplemental materials to promote understanding (stuffed animals, dolls).

- Suggest that the child help as much as possible; encourage the child to pretend and switch roles.
- Reinforce positive behavior with praise and rewards if necessary.
- Make sure you have obtained an accurate height and weight measurement.
- Be sure that you have compared the normal dose range with the dosage you plan to give; know toxic and lethal doses.
- Do not force medication on a frightened child, especially one who is crying.
- Always use two people when giving injections to small children.
- Disguise or dilute medications if necessary.

A nurse also needs to understand that the child's immature body systems may respond differently to drugs, so there may be changes in an agent's absorption, distribution, biotransformation, and elimination. (See Appendix F for information about pediatric intramuscular injections.)

Nursing Concerns for Geriatric Drug Administration

As with pediatric medications, special consideration is given when administering drugs to anyone who is over 65 years. This is because physiological changes caused by aging change the way the body reacts to certain drugs. For example, a tranquilizer may increase restlessness and agitation in an elderly person.

You should be aware of the following general considerations before administering a drug to any elderly individual.

- Small, frail elderly individuals will probably require less than the normal adult dosages. Drug absorption and distribution are affected by decreased gastrointestinal motility, decreased muscle mass, and diminished tissue perfusion.
- A drug should be given orally rather than parenterally, if possible, because decreased activity in the elderly decreases muscle tissue absorption.
- Often it will be necessary to crush pills, empty capsules, or dissolve medications in liquid in order to assist the person to swallow without discomfort. Tell patient *not to crush* enteric-coated or time-released drugs.
- Sedatives and narcotics must be given with extreme caution to elderly people, for they may easily become oversedated.
- Since the elderly are often on many different medications, you should check for drug interactions that may cause hazardous effects (e.g., giving a sedative shortly after a tranquilizer).
- Be alert to the cumulative side effects of the drugs you are administering. A drug's excretion may be altered if the patient has reduced renal blood flow and reduced kidney function.
- A schedule for rotation of injection sites should be followed carefully because the elderly have decreased muscle mass and increased vascular fragility.

- Any written directions for medication administration should be clear and in large print because of possible impaired vision.
- Be alert to the problem of impaired hearing when giving directions or asking questions. You may have to speak very loudly or repeat the same information several times. Writing the directions is recommended for some patients.
- Reinforce any important information by asking the patient to repeat it for you. This also helps you to ascertain that the information was understood. Memory loss and confusion are common in the elderly because of cerebral arteriosclerosis.

End of Chapter Review

Solve the following problems using Fried's rule.

1. The physician prescribed Spectrobid for a 12-month-old. The medicine was to be given q 12 h. The normal adult dose is 400 mg every 12 hours. The child would receive _____ mg every 12 hours.

2. A physician prescribed Pen-Vee K for an 18-month-old. The medicine comes in a powder

for oral suspension, 250 mg/5 ml. The normal adult dose is 250 mg every 6 hours. The nurse would give _____ mg in _____ ml every 6 hours.

Solve the following problem using Young's rule:

3. The physician prescribed Benadryl for an 8-year-old to relieve itching from chicken pox. Benadryl comes in an elixir of 12.5 mg/5 ml. The normal adult dose is 25 mg every 12 hours as needed. The nurse should give _____ mg in _____ ml every 12 hours.

Solve the following problem using Clark's rule:

4. A physician prescribed Dimetane for a 30-pound 4-year-old. The drug comes as an elixir, 2 mg/5 ml. The normal adult dose is 4.0 mg every 4 to 6 hours. The nurse would give _____ mg in _____ ml every 4 to 6 hours.

5. A physician prescribed Phenergan for a 45-pound child for preoperative medication. Phenergan is to be given as 1 mg/kg of body weight. The nurse would give _____ mg pre-operatively.

6. A physician prescribed tripelennamine hydrochloride for a 7-year-old who weighs 70 pounds and is 50 inches tall. The drug is to be administered as 150 mg/m^2/day in 4 equal doses. The normal adult dose is 50 mg every 6 hours. Refer to the nomogram in Figure 13–1 to find the child's surface area in square meters. Calculate the dosage the child should receive in four equally divided doses.

Chapter 14

Intravenous Therapies

Intravenous fluid therapy involves the administration of water, nutrients (dextrose, protein, fats, and vitamins), electrolytes (*e.g.*, sodium, potassium, chloride), blood products, and medications. Intravenous therapies are used in patients who need fluid replacement to treat disorders like dehydration, malnutrition, electrolyte imbalance, or tissue toxicity.

Intravenous hyperalimentation (total parenteral nutrition) is used for patients who cannot ingest food orally and are in a state of *negative nitrogen balance*. Intravenous hyperalimentation provides 1.0 to 1.5 gm of protein/kg of body weight. It is administered through a large blood vessel (*e.g.*, subclavian vein). Partial parenteral nutrition, administered through a peripheral vein, is used when the dextrose concentration is < 10% and therapy is < 2 weeks. Fat emulsions (Intralipid®) provide a concentrated form of non-protein kilocalories (primarily unsaturated fatty acids) yielding about 1.1 kcal/ml. Fat emulsions should never be mixed with a dextrose-amino acid solution (fat emulsions will break down). A list of commonly prescribed intravenous fluids can be found in Table 14–1.

Table 14–1. Commonly Prescribed Intravenous
Fluids

FLUIDS	ABBREVIATIONS
0.9% Sodium chloride solution	NSS
0.45% Sodium chloride solution	1/2 NSS
0.25% Sodium chloride solution	1/4 NSS
5% Dextrose in water	5% D/W D5W
10% Dextrose in water	10% D/W D10W
5% Dextrose in 0.45% sodium chloride solution	D5 1/2
Dextrose with Ringer's lactate solution	D/RL
Ringer's solution	R
Lactated Ringer's solution	RL

Plasma volume expanders
  Dextran
  Albumin	

Hyperalimentation
  Total Parenteral
  Nutrition
  Partial Parenteral
  Nutrition
	TPN
	
	PPN

Fat Emulsions Intralipid	

A physician request for intravenous fluid therapy
must include: the type of solution; the quantity of
solution; the time period for administration; and,
in some institutions or areas (pediatrics), the milliliters per hour. Several sample physician re-
quests for intravenous therapy are:

- Administer 1000 ml of D5W at 125 ml/hr.

- Administer 1000 ml of 0.9% NSS every 12 hours for 2 days.
- Administer 500 ml of D10W at 83 cc/hr.
- Administer 100 ml of RL over 4 hours at 25 ml/hr.

Intravenous fluids are administered through primary, secondary, or piggyback sets. Nurses can regulate the flow rate by calculating drops per minute or milliliters per hour. Frequently intravenous therapy is regulated by electronic devices. A *controller* electronically regulates drop rate, whereas an *infusion pump* consistently exerts pressure against the tubing or the fluid. Both devices improve the accuracy of therapy.

Medications are administered via the intravenous route: when rapid delivery is required, when a drug that is irritating to the tissues needs to be diluted and given with little trauma, or when a drug needs to be administered over a specified period of time. Intravenous administration of medications is frequently monitored by electronic flow rate regulators. Sometimes a medication is prescribed by intravenous "push"—which means the drug is given directly into an existing intravenous infusion, a heparin lock, or a vein. A disadvantage to administering medications intravenously is that drug sensitivities can develop quickly, and the medications given cannot be rapidly eliminated from the body.

Calculating Drops per Minute

■ **RULE: To Calculate Drops per Minute Use this Formula:**

$$\frac{\text{total amount of volume in ml} \times \text{drop factor*}}{\text{total time in minutes}}$$

$= \text{drops per minute (gtt/min)}$

EXAMPLE: Administer 1000 ml of D5W every 8 hours. The drop factor is 15 gtt/ml.

Use: $\qquad \dfrac{\text{total volume} \times \text{drop factor}}{\text{total time (minutes)}} = \text{gtt/min}$

$$\frac{1000 \text{ ml} \times 15}{480 \text{ min } (60 \times 8)} = \frac{15000}{480}$$

$= 31.25 \text{ gtt/min}$

Round off to 31.

Answer = 31 gtt/min

EXAMPLE: Administer 500 cc of 0.9% NSS over 6 hours. The drop factor is 20 gtt/ml.

Use: $\qquad \dfrac{\text{total volume} \times \text{drop factor}}{\text{total time (minutes)}} = \text{gtt/min}$

$$\frac{500 \times 20}{360} = \frac{10000}{360} = 27.7 \text{ gtt/min}$$

Round off to 28 gtt/min.

Answer = 28 gtt/min

* Check tubing package—may be 10, 15, 20 (macrodrip) 50, 60 (microdrip).

EXAMPLE: Administer 100 ml of an antibiotic solution over 60 minutes every 6 hours.
The drop factor is 60 gtt/ml.

Use: $$\frac{\text{total volume} \times \text{drop factor}}{\text{total time (minutes)}} = \text{gtt/min}$$

$$\frac{100 \times 60}{60} = \frac{6000}{60} = 100 \text{ gtt/min}$$

Answer = 100 gtt/min

Calculating Milliliters per Hour

■ **RULE: To Calculate Milliliters per Hour Use This Formula:**

$$\frac{\text{total volume}}{\text{total time (hours)}} = \text{milliliters per hour}$$

EXAMPLE: A patient is to receive 1000 ml of lac-
tated Ringer's solution over a 6 hour
period. The patient would receive
_____ ml/hour.

Use: $$\frac{\text{total volume}}{\text{total time (hours)}} = \text{milliliters}$$
per hour

$$\frac{1000 \text{ ml}}{6} = 166.6 \text{ ml/hr}$$

Round off to 167 ml/hour.

Answer = 167 ml/hour

End of Chapter Review

1. Administer 1000 ml of 0.9% NSS over 8 hours. The drop factor is 10 drops/ml. The flow rate would be _____ gtt/minute.

2. Administer 500 ml of D5W over a 12-hour period as KVO. The microdrip provides 60 drops per ml. The flow rate would be _____ gtts/minute.

3. To administer 1.0 liters of Ringer's lactate over 6 hours, you would give _____ ml/hour. The drop factor is 20 drops/ml.

4. The physician prescribed 1000 ml of D5W to infuse over 24 hours. With a drop factor of 15 gtts/ml, you would give _____ gtts/minute.

5. The physician prescribed 1000 ml of D5/0.9% NSS to infuse at 75 ml/hr. The drop factor is 15 gtts/ml. You would give _____ gtts/minute.

6. Ringer's lactate, 500 ml, is to infuse at 50 ml/hr. The drop factor is 10. You would set the rate at _____ gtts/minute.

7. To deliver 1000 ml of D5/0.45% NSS over 4 hours, the nurse would have to administer _____ ml/hr.

8. To deliver 500 ml of D5W over an 8-hour period, the nurse would set the flow rate to deliver _____ ml/hr.

9. To deliver 250 ml of NSS over a 5-hour period, the nurse would set the flow rate to deliver _____ ml/hr.

10. A patient is to receive 500 ml of 0.45% NSS with 20 mEq of KCL to run over 8 hours. The drop factor is 20 gtts/ml. The nurse would give _____ ml/hr.

11. The physician prescribed 100 ml of Albumin to be absorbed over 2 hours. The drop factor is 15 gtts/ml. The nurse would run the IV at _____ gtts/minute.

12. A patient is to receive 1000 ml of NSS with 20,000 units of Heparin over 24 hours. The drop factor is 60 gtts/ml. The nurse would give _____ gtts/minute.

13. A patient is to receive 350 mg of aminophylline in 150 ml of D5W over a 1-hour period of time. The drop factor is 15 drops per ml. The nurse would give _____ gtts/minute.

14. Administer 100 ml of an antibiotic solution via a volume control set over 30 minutes. The microdrip provides 60 drops per ml. You would give _____ gtt/minute.

15. A child is to receive 30 ml of an intravenous solution every hour through a volume control set that delivers 60 minidrops/ml. The flow rate should be set at _____ gtt/minute to deliver 30 ml/hour.

16. A hypertensive patient weighs 165 pounds. His physician prescribed Nipride 3 mcg/kg/ minute, IV. To administer, 50 mg of Nipride has to be added to a 250 ml solution of D5W. This solution would contain a concentration of Nipride, _____ mcg/ml. Using an infusion pump, the nurse would set the flow rate at _____ ml/hr.

17. The physician prescribed Mithracin 25 mcg/ kg by slow IV infusion for a patient who weighs 154 pounds. Mithracin is available in a vial labeled 2.5 mg/ml. To prepare the correct dose the nurse would add _____ ml of Mithracin to 1000 ml of D5W.

18. A patient is to receive Nitrostat 20 mcg/ minute IV. Nitrostat is available in a 10-ml vial labeled 5 mg/ml. To prepare a 40 mcg/ml solution, the nurse would add _____ ml of Nitrostat to a 250 ml D5W IV bottle, and then would set the infusion pump flow rate at _____ ml/hr to deliver 20 mcg/minute.

19. The physician prescribed 500 ml of a 10% Intralipid solution to infuse over 4 hours. Using a controller, the nurse would set the rate at _____ ml/hr.

20. The patient is to receive 150 mg of Dilantin by slow IV push for status epilepticus. Dilantin is labeled 50 mg/ml. The nurse would give _____ ml over a 10-minute period.

Chapter 15

Solutions

Solutions are mixtures of liquids, solids, or gases (known as *solutes*) that are dissolved in a dilutent (known as a *solvent*). Solutions can be administered externally (compresses, soaks, baths) or internally (irrigations, lavages), and they are usually prepared by a pharmacist or packaged by a pharmaceutical company. However, the preparation of solutions may increasingly become a nurse's responsibility as nursing's role outside the hospital institution expands to the home health care arena.

Solutions can be prepared from full-strength drugs or from stock solutions. Full-strength drugs are considered to be 100% pure, whereas stock solutions contain drugs in a given solution strength, always less than 100%, from which weaker solutions are made. Solution strengths can be expressed in a percentage or ratio format.

Solution problems are basically problems involving percents that can be solved using ratio-proportion. When setting up the ratio-proportion for a solution made from a pure drug or from a stock solution, *use the strength of the desired solution to the strength of the available solution as one ratio, and the solute to the solution as the other ratio.* Look at the proportion below:

desired solution strength: available solution
  strength
:: amount of solute: total amount of solution.

You can substitute an abbreviated formula when using a proportion for a solution made from a stock solution:

$$\frac{\text{desired strength}}{\text{on-hand strength}} \times \text{total amount of solution}$$

$$= \text{amount of solute needed}$$

When calculating solution problems, it is important to remember two things:

1. Work within the same measurement system (milligrams with milliliters, grains with minims).
2. Change solutions expressed in the fraction or colon format to a percent (1:2 or 1/2 should be equal to 50%).

Preparing a Solution From a Solution or Pure Drug

EXAMPLE: Prepare 500 cc of a 5% boric acid solution from pure boric acid crystals.

Proportion: $\dfrac{\text{desired strength}}{\text{available strength*}}$

$$= \frac{\text{amount of solute}}{\text{total amount of solution}}$$

$$\frac{5.0\%}{100\%} = \frac{x}{500 \text{ cc}}$$

*Available strength for a full-strength or pure drug is always 100%.

$$\frac{5}{100} = \frac{x}{500} \qquad 100x = 2500$$

$$x = 2500 \div 100$$
$$= 25 \text{ grams*}$$

Answer = 25 grams; weigh and dissolve 25 grams in 500 cc of water.

EXAMPLE: Prepare 1.0 Liter of a 10% solution from a pure drug.

Proportion: $\dfrac{\text{desired strength}}{\text{available strength}}$

$$= \frac{\text{amount of solute}}{\text{total amount of solution}}$$

$$\frac{10\%}{100\%} = \frac{x}{1000 \text{ ml}}$$

$$\frac{10}{100} = \frac{x}{1000} \qquad 100x = 10,000$$

$$x = 10,000 \div 100$$
$$= 100 \text{ ml}$$

Answer = Measure 100 ml of pure drug and add 900 ml of water to prepare 1.0 liter of a 10% solution.

*Answer is in grams because the solid form of boric acid was used and the solution desired was expressed in metric units.

Preparing a Solution
From a Stock Solution

EXAMPLE: Prepare 250 ml of a 5.0% solution from a 50% solution.

Formula: $\dfrac{\text{desired strength}}{\text{on-hand strength}} \times$ total amount

of solution = amount of

solute needed

$$\frac{\cancel{5\%}}{\cancel{50.0\%}} \times \overset{5}{\cancel{250}} \text{ ml} = 25 \text{ ml}$$

of solute needed

Answer = Measure 25 ml of the 50% solution and add 200 ml of water to prepare 250 ml of a 5% solution.

End of Chapter Review

1. To prepare 400 ml of a 2% sodium bicarbonate solution from pure drug, you would need _____ grams of solute.

2. To make 1.5 L of a 5.0% solution from a 25% solution, you would need _____ ml of solute. Add _____ ml of water to make 1.5 L.

3. There is 500 ml of 40% magnesium sulfate solution available for a soak. To make a 30% solution, you would need _____ ml of solute. Add _____ ml of water to make 500 ml.

Answer Key

Chapter 1

Practice Problems

Pages 5-6

1. ss	4. x
2. iii	5. xv
3. vii	6. xxx
7. 6	10. 9
8. 2	11. 20
9. 5	12. 25

End of Chapter Review, pages 6-7

1. xxvii	11. 18
2. xxxii	12. 16
3. xvi	13. 1/2
4. iv	14. 9
5. viii	15. 7 1/2
6. x	16. 19
7. xii	17. 24
8. xxi	18. 14
9. xviii	19. 26
10. xxiv	20. 6

Chapter 2

Practice Problems

Page 9

1. $\dfrac{4\text{-N}}{5\text{-D}}$

2. $\dfrac{1\text{-N}}{2\text{-D}}$

3. $\dfrac{3\text{-N}}{8\text{-D}}$ 5. $\dfrac{7\text{-N}}{8\text{-D}}$

4. $\dfrac{4\text{-N}}{9\text{-D}}$ 6. $\dfrac{1\text{-N}}{6\text{-D}}$

Page 11

1/300, 1/150, 1/100, 1/75, 1/25,
1/12, 1/9, 1/7 and 1/3

Page 12

1. 7, 1/8   4. 23, 1/25
2. 9, 1/10   5. 4, 1/150
3. 4, 1/5

Pages 15–16

1. 69/12   6. 87/4
2. 55/8   7. 37/2
3. 43/5   8. 57/9
4. 136/9   9. 27/5
5. 98/3   10. 67/6

Pages 18–19

1. 7 1/2   6. 2 2/3
2. 6 5/6   7. 4 3/10
3. 7 5/9   8. 7 3/4
4. 6 6/11   9. 9 5/9
5. 7 1/2   10. 22 2/5

Pages 22–23

1. 12/20	6. 6/10
2. 20/40	7. 1/6
3. 2/4	8. 1/6
4. 5/8	9. 1/4
5. 3/5	10. 1/18

Page 25

1. 1/6	3. 1/9
2. 1/6	

Pages 34–35

1. 2 5/11	6. 3/7
2. 13/16	7. 4/9
3. 3 19/24	8. 13/30
4. 1 2/45	9. 19/36
5. 1 3/10	10. 5 16/21

Pages 40–42

1. 14/45	6. 6 3/4
2. 5/21	7. 1 2/13
3. 3/20	8. 1 5/9
4. 1 7/20	9. 36
5. 21/32	10. 29/50

End of Chapter Review, pages 42–48

1. 14/35, 15/35
2. 28/20, 4/20
3. 1/6
4. 1/8
5. 6 1/2
6. 13 1/8
7. 50/11
8. 209/23
9. 5/16
10. 1/8
11. 1/9
12. 8/9
13. 1 1/3
14. 31/36
15. 7 5/24

16. 1/6
17. 5/9
18. 7/12
19. 4 9/40
20. 2 1/8
21. 3/20
22. 3/11
23. 14
24. 8
25. 6/11
26. 1 5/7
27. 24
28. 10 4/15
29. 5/56
30. 80

Chapter 3

Practice Problems

Pages 51–52

1. ten and one thousandths
2. three and seven ten-thousandths
3. eighty-three thousandths
4. one hundred fifty-three thousandths
5. thirty-six and sixty-seven ten-thousandths
6. one hundred twenty-five ten-thousandths

7. one hundred twenty-five and twenty-five-thousandths
8. twenty and seventy-five thousandths

Pages 52–53

9. 5.037
10. 64.07
11. 0.020
12. 0.4

13. 8.064
14. 33.7
15. 0.015
16. 0.1

Page 60

1. 38.2

2. 18.409

Page 61

3. 84.641
4. 243.58
5. 51.06

6. 12.33
7. 22.506
8. 6.8085

Page 62

9. 101.407
10. 1065
11. 70.88

12. 30.538
13. 0.0984
14. 0.0008

Pages 65–66

1. 0.20
2. 0.125
3. 0.25

4. 0.066
5. 0.066

Pages 66–67

6. 7/1000	9. 5 3/100
7. 93/100	10. 12 1/5
8. 103/250	

End of Chapter Review, pages 67–70

1. five and four hundredths
2. ten and sixty-five hundredths
3. eight thousandths
4. 6.08
5. 124.3
6. 16.001
7. 24.45
8. 59.262
9. 2.776
10. 5.210
11. 224.515
12. 0.1278
13. 1.56
14. 5.35
15. 0.60
16. 0.40
17. 0.142
18. 9/20
19. 6 4/5
20. 3/4

Chapter Four

Practice Problems

Page 75

1.	3/20	7.	33 1/3%
2.	3/10	8.	66.6%
3.	1/2	9.	20%
4.	3/4	10.	75%
5.	1/4	11.	40%
6.	3/5	12.	25%

Pages 77–78

1.	0.15	5.	25%
2.	0.25	6.	45%
3.	0.50	7.	60%
4.	0.80	8.	85%

Page 80

1. $\dfrac{50 \text{ milligrams}}{5 \text{ milliliters}}$ 50 mg:5 ml   50 mg/5 ml

2. $\dfrac{325 \text{ milligrams}}{1 \text{ tablet}}$ 325 mg:1 tab

   325 mg/1 tab

3. $\dfrac{2 \text{ ampules}}{1 \text{ Liter}}$ 2 amps:1 L   2 amp/1 L

Page 81

4. $\dfrac{1 \text{ tablet}}{5 \text{ grains}} : \dfrac{3 \text{ tablets}}{15 \text{ grains}}$

   1 tab:5 gr::3 tabs:15 gr

5. $\dfrac{0.2 \text{ milligrams}}{1 \text{ tablet}} : \dfrac{0.4 \text{ milligrams}}{2 \text{ tablets}}$

   0.2 mg:1 tab::0.4 mg:2 tabs

6. $\dfrac{10 \text{ milligrams}}{5 \text{ milliliters}} : \dfrac{30 \text{ milligrams}}{15 \text{ milliliters}}$

   10 mg:5 ml::30 mg:15 ml

Pages 85–86

1. 0.2 ml   3. 2 tablets
2. 3 tablets

End of Chapter Review, pages 86–89

Percent	Fraction	Decimal
1. 16.6%	1/6	0.166
2. 25%	1/4	0.25
3. 6.4%	8/125	0.064
4. 21%	21/100	0.21
5. 40%	2/5	0.40
6. 162%	1 31/50	1.62

Percent	Fraction	Decimal
7. 27%	27/100	0.27
8. 5 1/4%	21/400	0.052
9. 450%	9/2	4.50
10. 8 1/3%	1/12	0.083
11. 31%	31/100	0.31
12. 85.7%	6/7	0.857
13. 450%	18/4	4.5
14. 150%	1 1/2	1.5
15. 72%	18/25	0.72

16. $\dfrac{10 \text{ mg}}{1 \text{ tab}}$ 10 mg/tab

17. $\dfrac{10 \text{ units}}{1 \text{ ml}}$ 10 units/ml

18. $\dfrac{200 \text{ mg}}{1 \text{ kilogram}}$ 200 mg/kg

19. $\dfrac{100 \text{ mg}}{1 \text{ tab}} :: \dfrac{300 \text{ mg}}{x \text{ tab}}$

   100 mg:1 tab::300 mg:x tab

20. $\dfrac{250 \text{ mg}}{1 \text{ tab}} :: \dfrac{500 \text{ mg}}{x \text{ tab}}$

   250 mg:1 tab::500 mg:x tab

21. $\dfrac{0.075 \text{ mg}}{1 \text{ tab}} :: \dfrac{0.15 \text{ mg}}{x \text{ tab}}$

   0.075 mg:1 tab::0.15 mg:x tab

22. 20 mg:1 ml::10 mg:x ml

    20 mg $\times$ x ml = 10 mg $\times$ 1 ml

    $$20x = 10$$

    $$\frac{\overset{1}{\cancel{20}x}}{\underset{2}{\cancel{20}}} = \frac{\overset{1}{\cancel{10}}}{\underset{1}{\cancel{20}}} \quad x = \frac{1}{2} \quad x = \frac{1}{2}\text{ml}$$

    Answer $= \dfrac{1}{2}$ ml

    Verify the answer:

    extremes

    20 mg:1 ml::10 mg: $\dfrac{1}{2}$(0.5) ml

    means

    20 mg $\times$ 0.5 ml = 10 mg $\times$ 1 ml

    $\left.\begin{array}{l} 20 \times 0.5 = 10 \\ 10 \times 1 \ \ = 10 \end{array}\right\}$ Sum products are equal

23. $\dfrac{50 \text{ mg}}{5 \text{ ml}} = \dfrac{25 \text{ mg}}{x \text{ ml}}$

    Cross-multiply:

    50 mg $\times$ x ml = 25 mg $\times$ 5 ml

    $$50x = 125$$

    $$\frac{\overset{1}{\cancel{50}x}}{\underset{2}{\cancel{50}}} = \frac{\overset{5}{\cancel{125}}}{\underset{1}{\cancel{50}}}$$

$$x = \frac{5}{2} = 2\frac{1}{2} \text{ml}$$

Answer = 2.5 ml

Verify the answer:

$$\frac{50 \text{ mg}}{5 \text{ ml}} = \frac{25 \text{ mg}}{2.5 \text{ ml}}$$

$$50 \times 2.5 = 125 \Big\rbrace \text{Sum products}$$
$$25 \times 5 = 125 \Big\rbrace \text{are equal}$$

24. 3.0 mg:1.0 ml :: 1.5 mg : x ml

3.0 mg $\times$ x ml = 1.5 mg $\times$ 1.0 ml

$$3x = 1.5$$

$$\frac{\overset{1}{\cancel{3}}x}{\underset{2}{\cancel{3}}} = \frac{\overset{1}{\cancel{1.5}}}{\underset{1}{\cancel{3}}} = \frac{1}{2}$$

$$x = \frac{1}{2}$$

Answer = $\frac{1}{2}$ ml

Verify the answer:

extremes

3.0 mg:1.0 ml :: 1.5 mg:0.5 ml
means

3.0 mg $\times$ 0.5 ml = 1.5 mg $\times$ 1.0 ml

$$3.0 \times 0.5 = 1.5$$
$$1.5 \times 1.0 = 1.5$$
Sum products are equal

Chapter 5

Practice Problems

Page 95

1. 0.0360 M
2. 41.6 dm
3. 0.08 cm
4. 0.002 M

Page 97

1. 0.003006 L
2. 61.7 ml
3. 900 ml
4. 64 mg
5. 1.0 g
6. 0.008 dg

End of Chapter Review, pages 98–99

1. 0.00743 M
2. 0.006 dm
3. 10,000 M
4. 6217 mm
5. 0.0164 dl
6. 0.047 L
7. 1000 cl
8. 569 ml
9. 0.0356 g
10. 30 cg
11. 50 mg
12. 930 mg
13. 0.1 mg
14. 2000 mcg
15. 0.001 mg

Chapter 6

End of Chapter Review, page 103

1. griii
2. ʒv
3. fʒviii
4. mx
5. mxxsṡ or 20 m
6. pt. v

7. 2
8. 960 m
9. 32
10. 1/2
11. 1
12. 2

Chapter 7

End of Chapter Review, page 109

1. 2 cups
2. 24 oz.
3. 3 oz.
4. 120 gtts.

5. 9 tsps.
6. 12 oz.
7. 1/2 pt.
8. 1 pt.

Chapter 8

Practice Problems

Pages 113–114

1. 48–60 milliliters
2. 45–48 minims
3. 8–10 milliliters
4. 0.30 milligrams
5. 24–30 grams

6. 1 ounce
7. gr 1/10
8. 1 quart
9. 1 kilogram

194 ■ **Answer Key**

End of Chapter Review, pages 114–116

1. 25 kilograms
2. 60 grams
3. 960–1060 milliliters
4. 4 inches
5. 1 teaspoon
6. 300–325 milligrams
7. 3 drops
8. 1/150 grains
9. 8 drams
10. 300 mcg or 0.3 mg
11. 1.8 grams
12. 2 ounces
13. 6 tablets

Chapter 9

Practice Problems

Pages 120–122

1. 4 tablets
2. 45 ml
3. 1/2 tablet
4. 10 ml
5. 3 tablets
6. 2 tablets
7. 18.75 ml
8. 1/2 tablet
9. 1/2 tablet
10. 1 1/2 tablet
11. 3 tablets
12. 12 ml

Pages 125–126

1. 15 ml
2. 10 ml
3. 1 tablet
4. 15 ml; 45 mg
5. 4 tablets
6. 1 tablet
7. 18.75 ml
8. 12.5 ml
9. 2 tablets
10. 4 tablets
11. 4 tablets
12. 8 or 10 ml
13. 2.5 tablets
14. 4 tablets
15. 2 tablets

End of Chapter Review, pages 127–128

1. 3 tablets	6. 2 tablets
2. 3 tablets	7. 1 ounce
3. 30 ml	8. 1 tablet
4. 4 tablets	9. 7.5 ml
5. 1 tablet	

Chapter 10

Practice Problems

Pages 133–134

1. 2 ml	4. 3 ml
2. 4 ml	5. 0.8 ml
3. 3 ml	

End of Chapter Review, pages 134—137

1. 2.5 ml	9. 1.25 ml
2. 0.4 ml	10. 1.0 ml
3. 0.75 ml	11. 0.8 ml
4. 0.7 ml	12. 1.8 ml
5. 3.0 ml	13. 1.8–2.0 ml
6. 0.6 ml	14. 3.0 ml
7. 0.75 ml	15. 0.5 ml
8. 0.75 ml	16. 0.1 ml

Chapter 11

End of Chapter Review, pages 147–149

1. 0.6 ml	7. 4.0 ml
2. 0.25 ml	8. 1.2 ml
3. 0.8 ml	9. 15 units
4. 0.6 ml	10. 50 units
5. 0.5 ml	11. 34 units; NPH
6. 2.5 ml	12. 3; 2 units

Chapter 12

End of Chapter Review, pages 150-152

1. 0.5 ml
2. 0.5 ml
3. 8.8 ml
4. 2.0 ml

5. 12.5 ml
6. 3.0 ml
7. 13.5 ml
8. 0.5 ml

Chapter 13

End of Chapter Review, pages 165-167

1. 32 mg
2. 30 mg in 0.6 ml
3. 10 mg in 4.0 ml
4. 0.8 mg in 2.0 ml
5. 20 mg
6. Surface area = $1.0\ m^2$
   29 mg divided into 4 equal doses of 7.25 mg
   every 6 hours

Chapter 14

End of Chapter Review, pages 173-175

1. 21 gtts/min.
2. 42 gtts/min.
3. 167 ml/hr.
4. 10 gtts/min.
5. 19 gtts/min.
6. 8 gtts/min.
7. 250 ml/hr.
8. 63 ml/hr.
9. 50 ml/hr.
10. 63 ml/hr.

11. 13 gtts/min.
12. 42 gtts/min.
13. 38 gtts/min.
14. 200 gtts/min.
15. 30 gtts/min.
16. 200 mcg/ml;
    7 ml/hr.
17. 0.7 ml
18. 2 ml; 30 ml/hr.
19. 125 ml
20. 3.0 ml

Chapter 15

End of Chapter Review, pages 179–180

1. 8 grams
2. 300 ml; 1200 ml
3. 375 ml; 125 ml

Appendix A

Rounding Off Decimals

■ RULE: **To Round Off Decimals Follow These Steps:**

- Determine the place that the decimal is to be "rounded off" to (tenths, hundredths). For example, let's round off 36.315 to the nearest hundredths.
- Bracket the number [ ] in the hundredths place (2 places to the right of the decimal). For 36.315 you would bracket the 1. Then 36.315 would look like this 36.3[1]5.
- Look at the number to the right of the bracket. For 36.3[1]5 that number would be 5.
- If the number to the right of the bracket is:
  - less than 5 (<5), then drop the number.
  - 5 or greater than 5 (≥5), then increase the bracketed number by 1.

For 36.3[1]5 increase the bracketed number [1] by 1. The rounded off number becomes 36.32.

EXAMPLE: 5.671   5.6[7]1
                       Look at number to the
                          right of [7].
                       The number is <5.
                       Leave [7] as is; drop 1.
                       [7] stays as [7].
              5.671   rounds off to 5.67.

Answer = 5.67

Appendix B

Intradermal Injections

The intradermal route is preferred for:

- small quantities of medication (0.1 ml–0.2 ml)
- nonirritating solutions that are slowly absorbed
- allergy testing

THE INTRADERMAL ROUTE
Use A tuberculin syringe
Inject Into dermis or upper layer of tissue under the outer layer of skin or epidermis. Make sure the bevel of the needle is up.
Angle 15 degrees ↑ 15°

Injection Technique

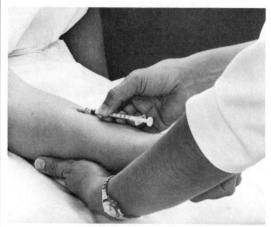

(From Wolff: Fundamentals of Nursing, 7th ed, p 691. Philadelphia, JP Lippincott, 1983)

Gauge		Needle Length		Solution	
Range	*Average*	*Range*	*Average*	*Range*	*Average*
27–25	26	$\frac{3}{8}-\frac{5}{8}$	$\frac{1}{2}$	0.1 ml–0.5 ml	0.1 ml

Appendix C

Subcutaneous Injections

THE SUBCUTANEOUS ROUTE

Use
- An insulin syringe
- A prefilled disposable syringe with
  appropriate needle length

Inject
  Under the skin into the fibrous tissue
  above the muscle

Angle*
  45–90 degrees

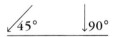

---

*A 45° angle of insertion is used with a 5/8″ needle for subcutaneous medications *except insulin and heparin;* for example, codeine sulfate and oxymorphone hydrochloride. A 90° angle of insertion is used with a 3/8″–1/2″ needle for *insulin and heparin*.

Injection Technique

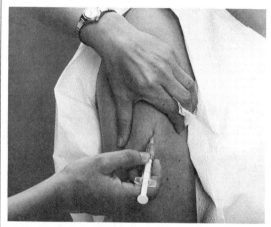

(From Wolff: Fundamentals of Nursing, 7th ed, p 693. Philadelphia, JP Lippincott, 1983)

Gauge		Needle Length		Solution	
Range	Average	Range	Average	Range	Average
27–25	25	$\frac{3}{8}-\frac{5}{8}$	$\frac{3}{8}-\frac{1}{2}$ $\bar{c}\ 90°$ $\frac{5}{8}$ $\bar{c}\ 45°$	0.2 ml– 2.0 ml	less than 1.0 ml

Appendix D

Intramuscular Injections

The *intramuscular route* is preferred for medications that:

- are irritating to subcutaneous tissue
- require a rapid rate of absorption
- can be administered in volumes up to 5.0 ml

THE INTRAMUSCULAR ROUTE
Use   A 3.0 ml–5.0 ml syringe
Inject   Into the body of a striated muscle. Inject past the dermis and subcutaneous tissue.
Angle   ↓ 90°   Always 90 degrees

Injection Technique

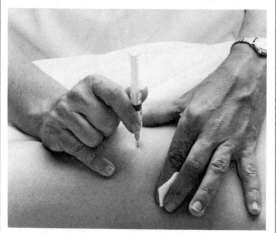

(From Wolff: Fundamentals of Nursing, 7th ed, p 697. Philadelphia, JP Lippincott, 1983)

Gauge		Needle Length		Solution	
Range	*Average*	*Range*	*Average*	*Range*	*Average*
25–20	22	1.0–2.0 inch	1.5 inch	0.5 ml– 5.0 ml	0.1 ml

Appendix E

Z-Track Injections

The *Z-track* method is used for parenteral drug administration when tissue damage from the leakage of irritating medications is expected, or when it is essential that all of the medication be absorbed in the muscle and not in the subcutaneous tissue. The method is easy, popular, and recommended by some institutions as a safe way of administering all intramuscular injections. This method prevents "tracking" of the medication along the path of the needle during insertion and removal.

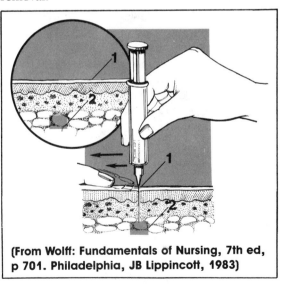

(From Wolff: Fundamentals of Nursing, 7th ed, p 701. Philadelphia, JB Lippincott, 1983)

THE Z-TRACK ROUTE

Use

A 3.0 ml–5.0 ml syringe

Inject

Deep into the body of the gluteal muscle; the vastus lateralis can also be used.

Angle

Always 90 degrees

↓ 90°

Injection Technique

Displace or push tissue over muscle toward the center of the body by displacing the tissue with the last three fingers of the nondominant hand. Hold the tissues in this displaced position before, during, and for 5 to 15 seconds after the injection so the medication can begin to be absorbed. Use IM injection technique as described on page 203.

Appendix F

Pediatric Intramuscular Injections

PEDIATRIC INTRAMUSCULAR INJECTIONS

Use

A needle about 1 inch in length. For infants a 5/8″ needle may be used.

Inject

Into dense muscle mass in the deltoid and ventrogluteal muscles. Into the outer quadrant of the gluteal and vastus lateralis muscles.

Angle

Preferably 45 degrees. May use 90 degrees if child's age and body mass warrant it.

Injection Technique

Similar to intramuscular technique for adults as described on page 203.

Gauge		Needle Length		Solution	
Range	Average	Range	Average	Range	Average
22–20	22	$\frac{1}{2}$–1.5 inch	1.0 inch	0.5 ml– 2.5 ml	0.5–1.0 < 3 years 0.5–1.5 4–6 yrs 0.5–2.0 7–14 yrs 1.0–2.5 > 15 yrs

Appendix G

Abbreviations and Symbols for Drug Preparation and Administration

ABBREVIATION/ SYMBOL	INTERPRETATION
a or ā	before
@	at
aa or $\overline{aa}$	of each
a.c.	before meals
A.D.	right ear
ad lib.	as desired
A.L. or A.S.	left ear
alt. h.	alternate hour
A.S.A.P.	as soon as possible
aq.	water
A.U.	both ears
b.i.d.	twice a day
b.i.n.	twice a night
c̄	with
C	gallon
cap(s).	capsule(s)
cc	cubic centimeter
cm	centimeter
comp.	compound
conc.	concentrate
D/C	discontinue
dil.	dilute
disp.	dispense
dist.	distilled
dr or ʒ	dram
Dx	diagnose

elix.	elixir
et	and
ext.	extract; external
fl; fld	fluid
g	gram
gal	gallon
Gm	gram
gr	grain
gtt	drops
h	hour
Ⓗ	hypodermic
h.s.	hour of sleep; at bedtime
ID	intradermal
IM	intramuscular
IV	intravenous
Kg	kilogram
KVO	keep vein open
L	liter
lb	pound
M; m	meter
m; min	minim
mcg	microgram
mEq	milliequivalent
mg; mgm	milligram
ml	milliliter
mm	millimeter
noct.	at night
N.P.O.	nothing by mouth
N.S.S	normal saline solution
O.	pint
o.d.; q.d.	once every day
O.D.	right eye
o.h.	every hour
O.S.	left eye
o.m.	every morning
o.n.	every night
OTC	over-the-counter
O.U.	both eyes
oz;ℨ	ounce
p̄	after
p.c.	after meals
per	by

p.o. or per os	by mouth
p.r.n.	as needed; when necessary
p.s.s	physiologic saline solution
pt	pint
q.	each; every
qh	every hour
q.i.d.	four times a day
q2h	every two hours
q3h	every three hours
q4h	every four hours
q6h	every six hours
q8h	every eight hours
q12h	every twelve hours
q.o.d.	every other day
q.s.	quantity sufficient; as much as needed
qt	quart
R	rectally
R/O	rule out
R_X	to take; by prescription
$\bar{s}$	without
s.c.; s.q.; sub.$\bar{q}$.; sub cut	subcutaneously
sig.	label; write
SL; subl.	sublingual
sol; soln	solution
s.o.s.	one dose as necessary
stat.	immediately
supp.	suppository
tab	tablet
tbsp; T	tablespoon
t.i.d.	three times a day
tinct; tr.	tincture
T.K.O.	to keep open
tsp; t	teaspoon
μg	microgram
ung.	ointment

Appendix H

Temperature Conversions: Fahrenheit and Celsius Scales

The Celsius scale is also known as the centigrade scale and is being used more often now that the metric system is becoming more popular. The Fahrenheit scale is used primarily for measuring body temperature.

- ■ RULE: **To Change From Fahrenheit to Celsius:**

  - Subtract 32 degrees from the Fahrenheit reading.
  - Multiply by 5/9.
  - $C = (F - 32) \times \dfrac{5}{9}$.

EXAMPLE: Convert 100°F to Celsius.

$$\begin{array}{r} 100 \\ -32 \\ \hline 68 \end{array} \quad \frac{68}{1} \times \frac{5}{9} = \frac{340}{9}$$
$$= 340 \div 9 = 37.7°C$$

Answer = 37.7° Celsius

- ■ RULE: **To Change From Celsius to Fahrenheit:**

  - Multiply Celsius reading by 9/5

- Add 32.
- F = (9/5 C) + 32.

EXAMPLE: Convert 40°C to Fahrenheit.

$$\overset{8}{\cancel{40}} \times \frac{9}{\underset{1}{\cancel{5}}} = 72 \quad \begin{array}{r} 72 \\ +32 \\ \hline 104° \end{array}$$

Answer = 104° Fahrenheit

You may find the temperature conversion scale shown here useful for quick reference.

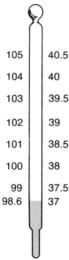

105	40.5
104	40
103	39.5
102	39
101	38.5
100	38
99	37.5
98.6	37

Water boils: 212° ⎫ Fahrenheit   Celsius ⎧ 100°: Water boils
Water freezes: 32° ⎭   ⎩ 0°: Water freezes

Temperature conversion scale

Index

Page numbers followed by *f* indicate figures; *n* following a page number indicates footnoted material; *t* following a page number indicates tabular material.